THE MAGIC POW]

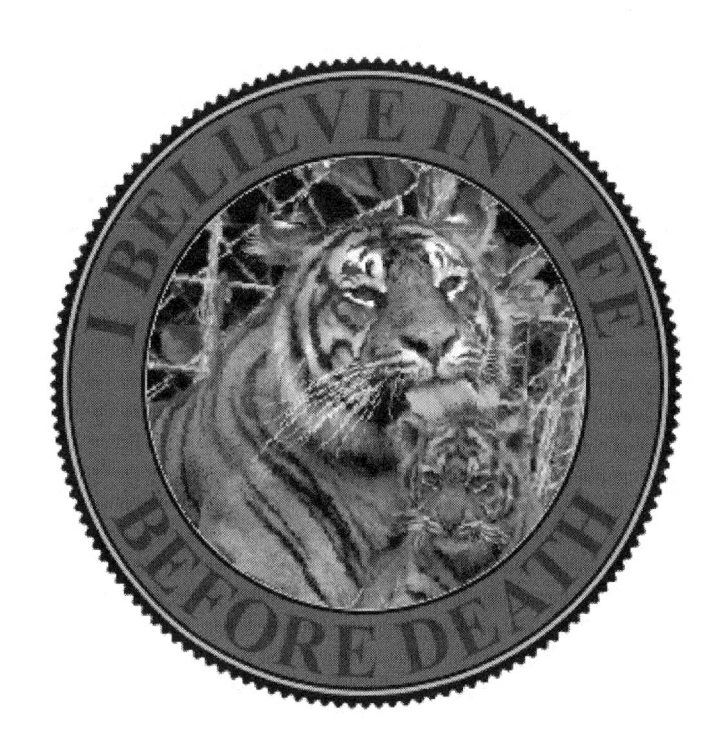

I AM THE TIGRESS

DEAN AMORY

Title: The Magic Power of Mental Images (I am the Tigress)

By: Dean Amory

Dean_Amory@hotmail.com

Publisher: Edgard Adriaens, Belgium

eddyadriaens@yahoo.com

ISBN: 978-1-291-42082-1

© Copyright 2013, Edgard Adriaens, Belgium, - All Rights Reserved.

This book contains contents of trainings, information found in other books and using the internet. A number of articles are indicated by TM or © or contain a reference to the original author. Whenever you cite such an article, please credit the source or check with the IP-owner. If you are aware of a copyright ownership that I have not identified or credited, please contact me at:

eddyadriaens@yahoo.com

Imagination is more powerful tan knowledge   (Albert Einstein)

INDEX

1. Definition and Use of Mental Imagery   13

1.1 What is Mental Imagery? 13
1.2 How do I use The Power of Mental Images 14
1.3 The Key To Achieving Your Goals 15
1.4 What is Visualization? 15
1.5 What Makes It Work? 16
1.6 How can I learn Mental Imagery 17
1.7 How to Implement Mental Imagery 17
1.8 Steps For Visualization: 18
1.9 Mental Imagery: Techniques 21

1. Manifesting Your Dreams and Desires *21*
2. Reducing Stress *22*
3. Shields, Safe Places and Mental Escapes *26*
4. Guided Imagery is about Goals *30*
5. Get rid of stumble blocks *30*
6. Autogenic Abreactions. *31*
7. Change with Covert Sensitization. *31*
8. Covert Behaviour Rehearsal. *31*
9. Problem Solving *32*
10. Clear Your Mind *33*
11. Balancing and centring *36*
12. Let Go and Break Free *36*

2. When, Why, How Use Mental Imagery?   40

2.1 Relaxation and Meditation 40

2.2 Building Confidence and Readiness 41
2.3 Preparing Success 42
2.4 Familiarizing 43
2.5 Doing a run-through. 44
2.6 Healing and Recovery 45
2.7 Behaviour Change 49
2.7 Behaviour Change 49

3. How To Develop Imagery Skills?   51

3.1 Imagery Categories 51
1. Motivational-specific (MS) *51*
2. Motivational general-mastery (MG-M) *51*
3. Motivational general-arousal (MG-A) *51*
4. Cognitive specific (CS) *52*
5. Cognitive general (CG) *52*
3.2 Where Do I Start? 52
1. Relaxation *52*
2. Realism *52*
3. Regularity *53*
4. Reinforcement *53*
3.3 Creating a Script 53
1. Basic picture *53*
2. Add details *53*
3. Refine the script *54*
4. Tape it *54*
5. Add more details *54*
6. Refine the script some more *55*

3.4 FITT 55
3.5 Practical Examples 57
3.5.1 How To Visualize Confidence *57*
3.5.2 Use Mental Imagery for Achieving Success *61*

4. Visioning   **75**

4.1 Introduction 75
4.2 Objectives: 75
4.3. Definition of Vision 75
4.4 How to discover your vision. 76
4.5 How to Create your success image 78
4.6 Visioning Techniques 79
4.7 Supplementary techniques 81
4.8 Take vitamins: 82
4.9. Managing The Visioning 83
1 Keep a log *83*
2 Keep your way *84*
4.10 Lesson summary 85
4.11 Do it yourself 86
4.12 Business Creativity 87
1 Introduction *87*
2 Objectives *87*
3. General Concepts *87*

5. Periscopic Learning aka Borrowed Genius   **103**

5.1 Steps: 104

6. How to Be Your Own Hero   **107**

6.1 "What do you want to be?" 107

6.2 The Seven Success Steps 109

7. Positive Affirmations   **111**

7.1 The importance of positive affirmations 111

7.2 Some words are better than others. 111

7.3 What are good words for you? 112

7.4 Free List of Positive Daily Affirmations 114

8. Animal Totems   **138**

8.1 I am the Tigress 138

8.2 Discover Your Personal Totem 140

8.3 Associations linked to some animals 141

9. Guided Imagery   **147**

9.1 What is Guided Imagery? 147

9.2 Guided Imagery Related to Stress Management 147

9.3 What is guided imagery used for? 148

9.4 Is guided imagery safe? 148

9.5 Example of a Free Relaxation Script 149

10. The Power of the Mind's Eye   **154**

10.1 See without seeing 154

10.2 Eyes Wide Shut: seeing with closed eyes 157

10.3 How mental images form in the brain 158

10.4 Mental representation 158

10.5 Mental imagery in experimental psychology 160

10.6 Training and learning styles 163

10.7 The Himalayan traditions 164

11. Healing Power and Visualization   **165**

11.1 Role of Imagination in Healing 165

11.2 Mental States and Physical Health 166

11.3 Case Studies 167

11.4 Summary 170

11.5 Wellness and Wholeness Visualizations 171

11.6 The Healing Power of the Mind 172

11.7 Define Your Specific Intention 174

11.8 How to Heal Yourself 177

11.9 Guided Imagery. 178

11.10 The Six Steps of Self Healing 179

12. Mental Imagery and Role Models   **181**

12.1 Objective of this Mental Strength Tip: 181

12.2 Modelling 181

12.3 Uncover Beliefs about Mental Thinking: 182

12.4 Unsupportive Beliefs about Role Models 182

12.5 Mental Strength Beliefs about Role Models 182

12.6 Outrageous Questions: 182

12.7 Reflective Questions: 182

12.8 Mental Strength Coaching: 182

12.9 Final Thought 183

12.10 Role models are important. 183

12.11 Focus on what is good.. 185

12.12 How To Choose The Right Role Model 185

12.13 How To Become Who You Want To Be 188

12.14 Examples. ...189
12.15 Four Common Mistakes ...190

13. How to Think Like a Genius   **194**

13.1 Steps ...195

14. Visualisation Boards   **199**

14.1 Personality Boards ...199
14.2 Vision Boards or Dream Boards ...202
14.3 The Power of Vision Boards ...203
14.4 Action Boards ...209
14.5 Throw Away Your Vision Board ...211

15. Powerful Words Evoke Powerful Images   **219**

15.1 The Power of Metaphors ...219
15.2 What is a metaphor? ...220
15.3 List of strong metaphors ...221
15.4 The power of metaphors ...224
15.5 Limitations of metaphors ...225
15.6 Metaphor is how we learn ...225
15.7 Where did you get your metaphors? ...226
15.8 Test this out for yourself. Your exercise: ...227
15.9 How metaphors work ...228
15.10 How metaphors influence ...231
15.11 Powerful Metaphor Communication ...232
15.12 The Metaphor of our lives: ...233

16. The Bucket List   236

16.1 What is a Bucket List? 236
16.2 Why Create A Bucket List? (from Celes) 237
16.3 How to Create Your Bucket List 238
16.4 101 items to consider for your bucket list. 240
16.5 After you finish your list: 245

17. The Power of Mental Imagery   247

17.1 HOW TO INFLUENCE OTHERS (CHAPTER III) 248
17.2 THE CREATIVE IMAGINATION (CHAPTER V) 251

1. Definition and Use of Mental Imagery

1.1 What is Mental Imagery?

Mental imagery, also called visualization and mental rehearsal, is defined as experience that resembles perceptual experience, but which occurs in the absence of the appropriate stimuli for the relevant perception.

Whenever we imagine ourselves performing an action in the absence of physical practice, we are said to be using imagery. While most discussions of imagery focus on the visual mode, there exists other modes of experience such as auditory and kinaesthetic that are just as important.

A mental image is a picture, scene or event that you see in your mind. You construct mental images in your mind all the time, albeit unconsciously. The mental images that you often visualize affect your life, whether you are aware of this or not. I am not talking mental images that you visualize once or twice, but about the mental images that you often repeat in your mind.

Mental images have the power to change your life. The subconscious mind accepts these images as reality, and gradually you start to believe what you imagine, act accordingly, and unconsciously work toward making them a reality in your life. This is the secret of the law of attraction creative visualization.

Mental images, if repeated often can make great changes in your life. If you visualize negative situations, difficulties and problem, and continue doing so, your moods will gradually become negative, you will alienate people, you will close your eyes to opportunities, and your self-esteem will go down. How can you achieve success if you are so negative?

On the other hand, successful people attract success, because they constantly imagine and expect success.

Mental images are like a movie or still pictures that you see in your mind. If you watch them again and again your subconscious mind will ultimately accept them as you reality. They will affect your thinking, behaviour and world.

1.2 How do I use The Power of Mental Images

The power of mental images can change your life if you use it consciously, and if learn to choose your mental images and reject those that are not good for you. You can decide what mental scenes you see in your mind. You can decide what to let seep into your subconscious mind.

Always be aware of your thoughts. When you catch yourself visualizing negative events, problems or difficulties, or when you tell yourself that you are helpless and weak, stop that and change the mental movie and the words you repeat in your mind. It is like ejecting a DVD from your DVD player and inserting a better and more interesting one.

Visualize what you really and truly desire, and what will make you happy and satisfied. Your mind will probably interfere with fears, worries and disbelief. Your job is to educate your mind and change its habits, and you can do so if you realize the power of mental images and use it correctly.

Being aware of your thoughts, replacing negative thoughts with positive thoughts, and visualizing positive mental images again and again, will eventually change the habits of your mind and your thinking. This will lead to understanding and realizing the power of mental images.

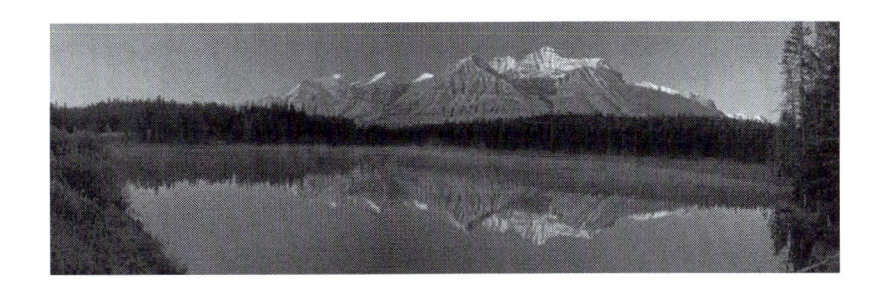

1.3 The Key To Achieving Your Goals

Visualization is an important personal development tool. Just as affirmations can help you motivate yourself and focus better to achieve your goals so can using visualization or mental imagery.

Whenever we have an idea or notion to do something we visualize it first. For instance, if we're hungry and want to eat we picture different food possibilities; whether we want to cook a meal or go out to eat, and whether or not we want company at our meal. When we have a function to attend we picture what type of outfit to wear and where we might shop for it.

1.4 What is Visualization?

It is the use of the imagination through pictures or mental imagery to create visions of what we want in our lives and how to make them happen. Along with focus and emotion it becomes a powerful, creative tool that helps us achieve what we want in life.

Used correctly it can bring about self-improvement, maintain good health, help you perform well in sports, and accomplish your goals in life.

In sports, mental imagery is often used by athletes to improve their skills by picturing the achievement of a specific feat, such as hitting or shooting a ball, skiing a hill, swimming or running a race, among other things.

Using it as a technique invariably results in a much better performance and outcome. This also holds true in business or in life such as in delivering a speech, asking for a raise or any other situation that requires preparedness and forethought.

1.5 What Makes It Work?

Visualization or mental imagery works because when you imagine yourself performing perfectly and doing exactly what you want, you physiologically create neural patterns in your brain, just as if you had physically performed the action. The thought can stimulate the nervous system in the same way as the actual event does.

Performing or rehearsing an event in the mind trains it and creates the neural patterns to teach our muscles to do exactly what we want them to do.

In the case of competitive sports, not only are exceptional physical skills required, but so is a strong mental game. Most coaches preach that sports are 90% mental and only 10% physical. That's why so many athletes train in visualization or mental imagery along with their physical routines.

To be effective, like any skill, mental imagery needs to be practiced regularly. The four elements to mental imagery are relaxation, realism, regularity and reinforcement.

Creative visualization is a very useful way to contribute to successful goal achievement. In this procedure you use your imagination to create a clear picture in your mind of whatever you want to take place in your life.

1.6 How can I learn Mental Imagery

Virtually everyone can successfully use imagery. It's a question of patience and persistence. It's just like learning to play a music instrument or learning to fly an airplane. You put in the time, you put in the discipline, you will be able to do it. It is the same with imagery.

Practice, practice and practice. You will be able to do it.

How much time it will take before you begin to see results depends on the severity of your ailment, the vividness of your imagery and your own determination. A person who has a sprained ankle, for example, may get pain relief in just one five-minute imagery session, while it may take weeks for a person who has severe burns to notice any significant pain reduction. For almost any chronic ailment, it's going to take a lot more time for imagery to work.

Most proponents suggest practicing your imagery for 15 to 20 minutes a day initially to ensure that you're learning to do it properly. But as you become more skilled and comfortable with the technique, you'll be able to do it for just a few minutes at a time as needed throughout the day.

1.7 How to Implement Mental Imagery

There is no correct way to practice mental imagery. It is all left up to individual preferences and the present circumstances. It can be done "on or off the field", very short (within a few seconds or minutes) or of a long duration; sitting up, lying down, in complete silence, with a stereo, eyes closed or open.

A shorter version of imagery is best implemented during match play or while executing a task. For example, a tennis player may take a few seconds to visualize him or herself hitting the perfect serve in the place where he or she wants. Or a quarterback can go through a play in his mind just before calling the play.

Longer, specific guided visualizations are usually designed for a quiet room prior to meeting a challenge, e.g. competition. In this case, the player should be in a relaxed and receptive state in order for the image to go deeply into the mind.

It is recommended to do visualization two or three times per week.

Another way that many athletes practice imagery is during bike rides, lifting weights, rowing, etc. Since one is exerting physical energy while doing mental rehearsal, it helps facilitate actual competition (Porter, 22-23).

Some individuals are better at forming pictures in their heads than others. Or some people may excel in certain sensory experiences and not others. Advice on improving mental imagery skill can be found

1.8 Steps For Visualization:

Studies indicate that mental imagery works best when it is used in conjunction with a relaxation technique. When your physical body is relaxed, you don't need to be in such conscious control of your mind, and you can give it the freedom to daydream. Meditation, progressive relaxation or yoga are the most common relaxation techniques used with mental imagery.

1. Go to a place where you will be undisturbed.

2. Sit in a comfortable chair. Loosen your clothing, take off your shoes, and sit comfortably. You can also use one of the yoga or meditation postures. Dim the lights, if you prefer.

You might want to put some music on to stimulate your right brain (the creative and feeling part of you which can help you draw on the power of your unconscious to move invisible energy towards your desired goal).

You might like to explore the use of aromatherapy oils. They can be worn or burned in a special burner to gently fill the air and stimulate the senses to create positive and soothing feelings, which can greatly enhance the power of visualizations.

3. Close your eyes and relax. Take in a few deep breaths. Breathe in and out slowly for 10 times to attain maximum relaxation.

4. Start to see in your mind's eye, the thing you want, in as much detail as possible (as you practice and get better at visualizations, see if you can make the picture brightly colored, sharply focused, framed, containing sound, action and feeling).

5. Step into the picture and energize it with 5 big breaths.

6. Make an affirmation sub-vocally, to put the event in present tense and make it real. Gain the feeling of actually achieving what you want. Say to yourself, "This is mine, right now!".

You might like to vary your visual pictures, depending on your mood. Some people love the visual picture of being on a beach; others prefer the mountains in a snowstorm! Use your imagination and treat yourself to visualizations that bring you maximum relaxation and positive feeling.

It's important to visualize with as much detail and using as many senses as possible. For example, if you want a new car, specify the kind in detail, see yourself driving the car, feel the steering wheel and be aware of the instrument panel, the texture of the seats and everything else about it that you want.

Visualization should be done regularly and may be consistently reinforced if done either first thing in the morning or last thing at night. You may wish to make your own audiotape. If you don't like your own voice, ask someone else to make a tape for you.

Visualization is a powerful process and can overcome past negative programming.

It's time to relax and enjoy the mental creation of your goals. In taking that short time to relax and trust that your right brain is doing the hard work, you will find that the benefits are that when you return to this manual, your mind will be more alert, clear, and the flow of good ideas should come more easily.

7. Just before you want to end your session, take a few more deep breaths and picture yourself re-climbing the imaginary staircase and gradually becoming aware of your surroundings. Open your eyes, stretch, smile and go on with your day.

Sources:

Achieve Your GOALS - The Complete Goal Management System - INFORMATION AND EDUCATION SERVICES
www.thepdi.com   -   www.thepdi.com/donaldcarty

© Copyright 2005 Personal Development Institute Atlanta, Georgia 30518, USA

http://www.nursingstudentsupport.net/content/SAPDF/SM20.Mental Imagery.pdf

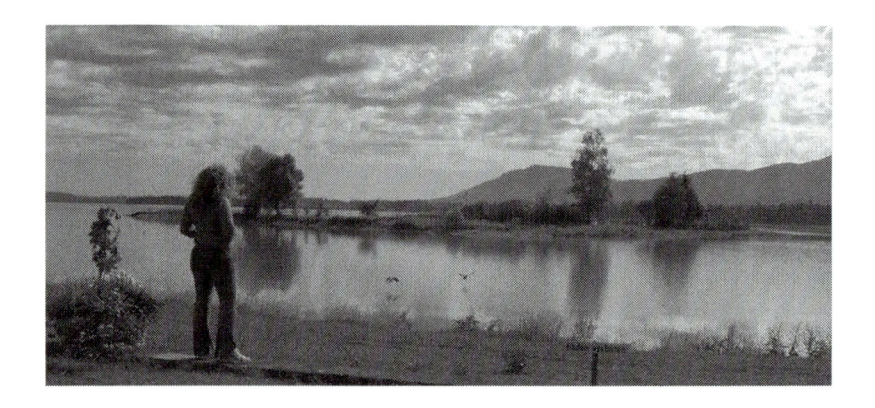

1.9 Mental Imagery: Techniques

Several different types of imagery are used depending on the application and desired result. Most visualization techniques begin with relaxation, followed by summoning up a mental image.

If you can imagine it, you can create it in your life. Visualizations are mental images that can help us to leap over obstacles, shrink our troubles, manifest our dreams, reduce our stresses, let go of regrets, and invent new ideas. Visualization is also an excellent decision-making tool.

You have the freedom of choosing the type of pictures you want to focus on, depending on your intent.

Take this visual tour to discover a variety of purposes for using visualization.

1. Manifesting Your Dreams and Desires

(By Phylameana lila Desy, About.com Guide)

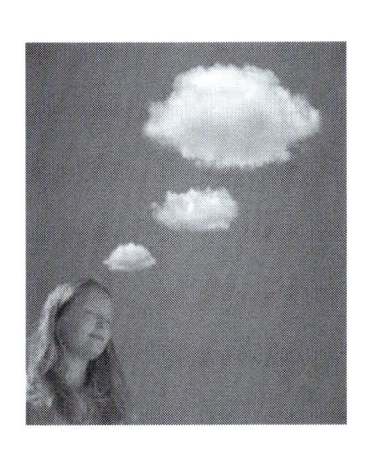

Has the power of visualization or law of attraction alluded you because you have no idea what it is you want? Not having a clear idea of what you want you want can certainly be a stumbling block in attracting any good stuff. Dreams do come true, but first you have to dream them, Right? Not to worry, it is okay to be clueless from time to time. It just might be that you are content with your life as it is right now, or, you may truly feel as if you are in too dark of a place psychologically right now. Everyone knows how feelings of sadness or despair can create a shadow of any glimmer of hope. You may feel that it is difficult or even impossible to formulate a picture in your head of your desires when you don't have a clue.

The Key to Unlocking Your Dreams Visualization

This lock and key visualization exercise can be used whenever you don't have anything specific you'd like focus on. Imagine a key and a lock in your mind. Think of the lock as the place where all your dreams are hidden from view. Consider the key as a tool for unlocking your dreams.

Simply visualize both the key and the lock side by side, then as you deepen your visualization imagine that the key is in your hand with you preparing to insert the key into the keyhole. Visualize unlocking the lock with a turn of the key. That's it. Continue practicing this simple key visualization routinely. The exercise of visualizing "unlocking" the lock over and over again will help you become a pro at the art of visualization.

Overtime, you can begin adding additional elements into your visualization. You could incorporate a light beam, doorway, or pathway to help show you the way. Later on try transforming the lock into a treasure chest filled with golden coins and precious gems, or a trunk with beautiful wedding gown tucked inside, or try unlocking a roll top desk with a rolled college diploma stashed into a cubbyhole.

2. Reducing Stress

Stress is a huge problem for so many people. We are overwhelmed on a daily basis because of having too many responsibilities. So many tasks to tend to and hardly any rest for the weary. Purging or releasing visualizations are intended to tackle those stresses head on and squash them like bugs. It is important to make de-stressing a priority exercise.

- To reduce stress, try concentrating first on a colour you associate with tension, and then mentally replace it with one that you find soothing; for example the colour red changing to blue.

- Or you may find it more relaxing to picture a peaceful natural scene, such as the unruffled surface of a pond, gently rolling hills, a serene waterfall, evening in a beach watching the sun set, etc.

- Still another technique is to picture yourself descending an imaginary staircase. With each step, you notice that you feel more and more relaxed.

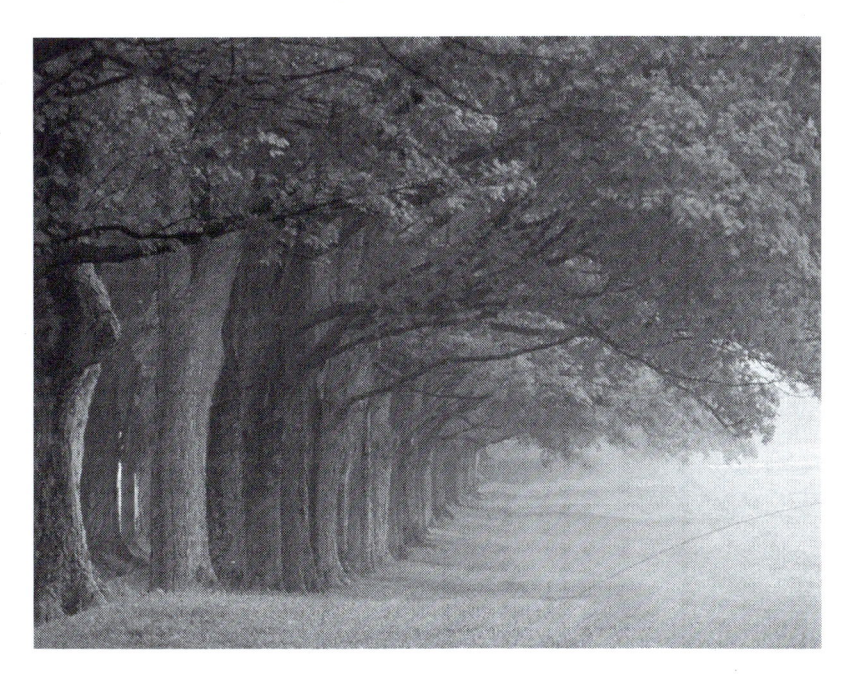

- Or you can float like the leaf of a tree, travel the waters of a lovely creek enjoying the summer breeze and the beautiful, peaceful meadows that you are passing through.

- Pull the Plug and Drain All Your Stresses Away (By Phylameana lila Desy, About.com Guide) Relaxing in the tub is wonderful way to end your day and wash away your stresses. While soaking in your bath imagine that all the "emotional gunk" and "mental crazies" of your day are being lifted from your mind and scrubbed off your body. Say "bye-bye" to these "undesirables" when you pull the plug. Watch all your troubles gurgle down the drain pipe along with your bath water. Good riddance! Make a deep sigh, put a smile on your face, step out of the empty tub, and pat yourself dry with a big fluffy towel. Taking a stress purging bath in the evening will also help you.

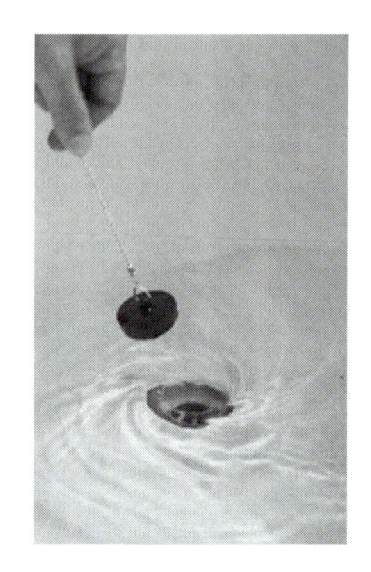

- Punching Bag Visualization (From Jackie) - I imagine whatever or whoever is the focus of my frustration is a punching bag, and then I let loose on it. Someone suggested that I either take a baseball bat to my mattress or join a gym and beat a punching bag with my fists as ways to take out my frustrations. But, I'm pretty much a wimp and figured if I broke a nail then I'd really be ticked off, so instead, because I am a visual creature I began doing what was suggested in the safe recesses of my mind.

Simply imagining slapping your snotty co-worker silly, punching your intimidating boss in the gut, or dumping a ton of bricks over your nosy brother-in-law's head can be a real trip. No blood or gore, only anger-releasing satisfaction.

Tips and Tricks

- Not everyone can vent their emotions through actions, this visualization is merely a substitute for meeker spirits.
- After your mental fight, take off your gloves and create a relaxing visual in your head.

- Painting: Close your eyes, cover them with your palms, and concentrate on the colour black. Try to make the colour fill your whole visual field, screening out any distracting images.

- Mountain Top Visualization (From Cathy) - I transport myself to a mountain top where I breathe away negativity easily and effortlessly. Parked close to the edge, I relax and deep breathe. On inspiration (inhalation) I gather any negativity together and on expiration (exhalation) I visualize breathing it out. I watch it go over the edge, flow onto jagged rocks into a body of water which is acid. The water dissolves all negativity, which will not reoccur.

As I repeat the breathing I visualize healing white light filling all the cells of my body. When I know that I am full of healing light I sit and rest.

Tips and Tricks

- I usually do this at night and I fall asleep and sleep soundly.
- Make the visualization yours with objects and thoughts that give you peace.
- Practice, practice, practice.

3. Shields, Safe Places and Mental Escapes

Visualization is a wonderful tool for periodic escapes from the mundane. No matter where you are physically you can train your mind to carry you away to a more exotic destination or a more comfortable place.

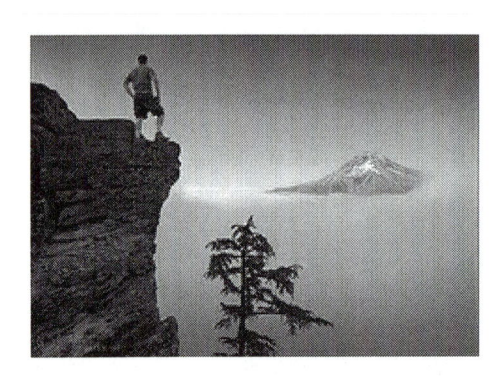

Daydreamers are superb at taking mental escapes. In fact, chronic daydreamers would be wise to train their wandering minds from floating away so often and learn to focus more on the reality of where they are.

Mental escapes are best used for "rest" or "relaxation" not for avoidance.

My mind has a habit of taking off to a visual world of my own making during commercial breaks whenever I'm watching a television program.

Advertisers won't like hearing this, but that's usually what happens: After I've seen a commercial once, my mind doesn't stick around when it is replayed over and over again. I'll make a preferred mini-movie within my own mind in its place. When the televised show comes back on, my mental retreat ebbs until the next commercial break. Weird, I know.

When you feel relaxed, imagine a favourite scene. It could be a beach, a mountain slope or a particularly enjoyable moment with friends or family.

Try to go into this scene each time you practice your visualisation-session. If you can create a special, safe place where nothing can hurt you and you feel secure, it will make you more receptive to other images. Once you feel comfortable in your favourite scene, gradually direct your mind toward the ailment you're concerned about.

Use an image that is very pleasant for you or allow your mind to create a different one of its own. Let the image become more vivid and in focus. Don't worry if it seems to fade in and out. If several images come to mind, choose one and stick with it for that session.

Beach Visualization: How to do it

(Simple Visualizations – Article From Paul B.)

- Find quiet place where you can lay down or recline in a lounger.
- Close your eyes and take a relaxing breath.
- In your mind paint a picture of beach with blue skies and deep blue green water.
- A few more mental brush strokes and you'll discover yourself sitting under a palm tree.
- Imagine the sounds of the water and smells of the salty air along with your visuals.
- You know you're doing good when you can almost feel the sand between your toes.

Shielding

These "protective" visualizations are meant to shield you from negativity and unwanted attacks. Humans are meant to interact with one another. Why else would we choose to incarnate into a physical body and live together, work together, and play together? However, the merging of too many energies may at times feel overwhelming, even frightening. Forming protective imagery in your visualizations in your mind can assist you in learning how to deflect negativity and to create clear boundaries.

Drawing a Line in the Sand

Whenever I feel my personal boundaries are at risk, I will mentally draw a line in the sand. This picture helps me feel more in control.

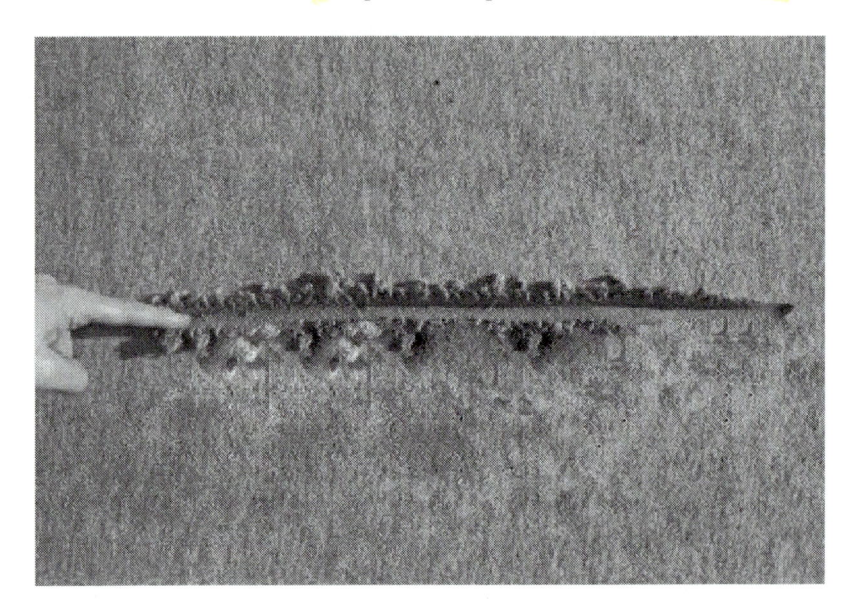

I mentally transport myself to a sandy coastline. Then, imagine myself stooping over and with my hand or fingers draw a line in the sand.

The line in the sand represents a safe boundary. No one can cross it, nor are you expected to go step over this line and do anything you are not comfortable with. You are basically creating boundaries. This visualization is helpful for anyone who has trouble saying no or feels badly when they refuse doing favours for others. The line in the sand gives you the strength to say no when someone is asking you to do something, also frees you of guilt.

Tips and Tricks

- Try drawing a circle in the sand with you safely inside. No one can sneak up on you from behind.

- When you are ready to broaden your safe area, imagine the ocean tides coming to shore and washing away your drawn line. Now move back and draw a new line that gives you more space.

Return to sender with love

Sandra Ingerman, author of How to Heal Toxic Thoughts, suggests deflecting harmful energies by using this intentional visualization. Similarly to refusing the delivery of an unwanted postal package by scribbling the words "Return to Sender" across the box, whenever you feel you are the target of negativity imagine the harmful energies locked safely inside an unopened box. Then visualize yourself writing the words "Return to Sender with Love" while infusing love energies into the container. Finally, imagine that you are dropping it into the nearest mailbox for pickup. Not only will you be sending the energies back to where they originated from, but you will have transformed the energies into loving vibrations. In this way you are protecting yourself from harm, defusing lethal toxicity, and refusing to exasperate a negative situation.

Tips and Tricks

If you have trouble visualizing try to think of your meditation as a blank canvas. You are the artist. Be your own creator.

Visualize the landscape that relaxes you best (beach, forest, mountains, desert oasis, etc.).

On the other hand, if no visual images come to mind, try focusing on a different sensation. For instance, imagine hearing fish frying in a skillet or smelling wild flowers in a meadow.

If all else fails, think about how you feel at the moment. Angry? Frustrated? What colour is that anger? What image is evoked? Use these feelings to forge images. Each time you do this, imagine that your ailment will be completely cured / goal will be reached at the end of the session.

4. Guided Imagery is about Goals

Define priorities, visualize your goals and imagine how you will achieve them.

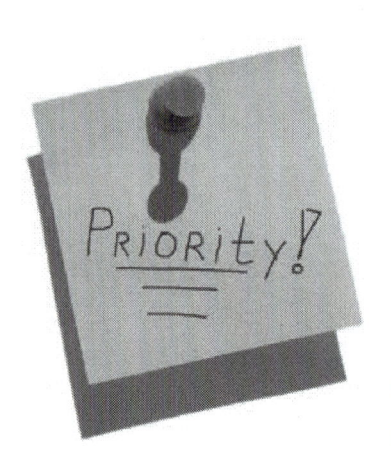

In this technique, participants visualize a goal they want to achieve, then imagine themselves going through the process of achieving it.

Severely ill patients, for example, are urged to picture their internal organs and imagine them free of disease, or to picture tumours shrinking, or invading micro-organisms succumbing to aggressive immune cells.

5. Get rid of stumble blocks

Eliminate irrational believes, fear and internal conflicts with Guided Waking Imagery.

In this technique, devised by the psychoanalyst Leuner, the patient it taught to visualize a standard series of scenes such as a meadow, a mountain, a house, and a swamp.

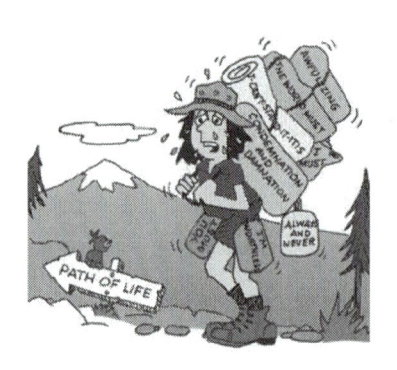

Later, the patient's imaginings are examined for sources of conflict, irrational beliefs, and interpersonal problems.

6. Autogenic Abreactions.

Assume an attitude of passive acceptance toward your mental experiences. In this condition, verbalize, without restriction, all the thoughts, feelings, and sensations that occur to you. Continue until the discharge has run its course. If strong affect emerges, often with marked emotional and facial involvement is likely to emerge. The session continues until the effective discharge has run its course.

7. Change with Covert Sensitization.

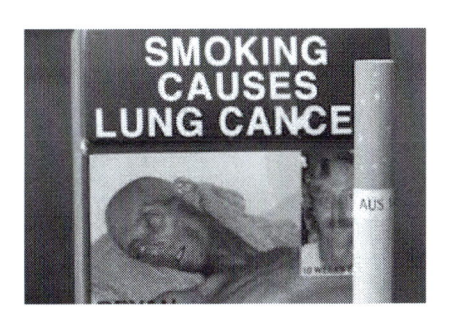

This technique is based on the reinforcement paradigm. It postulates that imagery processes can be modified according to the same principles that govern the modification of overt, visible behaviour. In covert sensitization, the patient first imagines engaging in some behaviour he wishes to change, say, an addiction. This is quickly followed by the imagining of a highly unpleasant event. Thus, the addictive behaviour becomes paired with a highly aversive event and therefore is less likely to occur in the future.

8. Covert Behaviour Rehearsal.

Improve your technique with Covert Behaviour Rehearsal

In this method, the individual systematically visualizes the desired correct coping behaviour. This technique has seen much use in sports.

9. Problem Solving

Are you facing difficulties in your life? Or are you challenged with making a decision? Visualization can help.

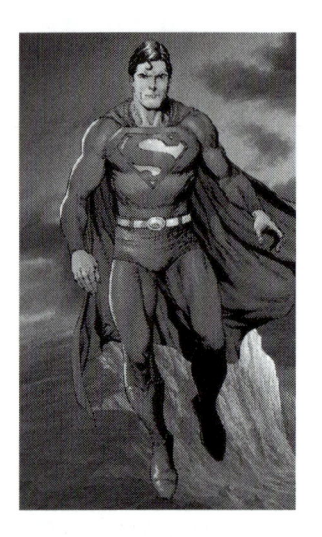

You can choose an image to focus on to help you through a troublesome period. Visualize yourself as a superwoman who can easily scale the highest skyscrapers or a marathon runner who outruns all of his competitors. Put your problems inside a carton and imagine it getting smaller and smaller until it can easily fit into your pocket. You'll discover that your problem is easier to carry inside your pocket than the heavy weight of it sitting on your shoulders. Or, you can visualize your problems magically disappearing before your eyes. There are no limitations in your visualizing. It can be magical.

When you are struggling with making a decision between two different options, try visualizing yourself involved in the two scenarios.

For example, let's say you are having trouble choosing between two different breeds of dogs to welcome into your family as your new pet.

Imagine taking each of the two dogs individually on walks or trips to the vet. Picture yourself grooming them, feeding them, playing with them, etc. Visualize how each dog will age, imagine it growing from a cute puppy into a full grown animal. Picture these two dogs living within your home and interacting with you and your family members. Hopefully this visualization exercise will help you in deciding the perfect dog breed to fit your life style.

You can do similar visualizations when choosing regions to live in, schools to attend, career option opportunities, etc. Even when confronted with an uncomplicated choice, such as choosing what colour to paint your bedroom, this can be decided through the help of visualization.

10. Clear Your Mind

Clearing Mental Clutter (By Phylameana lila Desy, About.com Guide)

Too many thoughts and mental pictures can convolute the mind. It may seem strange to use visualization to reduce the chaos in your brain when your mind already feels too crowded, but it can help. The idea is to choose images that erase, filter, or organize your thoughts. Much like de-cluttering a closet, you can use visualization to reduce mental clutter.

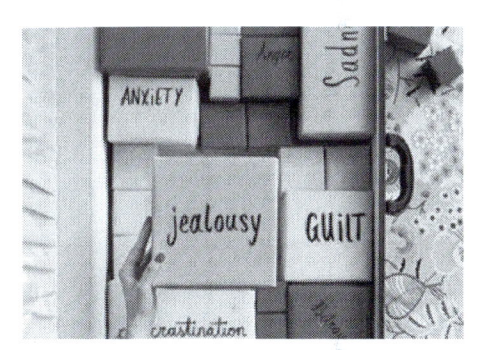

There are three causes of mental clutter: Avoidance, Indecision, and Procrastination

Do you have a mental "to-do list" that is overloading your brain power? Or is indecisiveness possibly robbing you of clear and focused thought?

A Case of Brain-Drain

Make an effort to periodically clear your mind of any obsessive thoughts that are overwhelming you. You will likely be bogged down with a serious case of brain drain unless you routinely take the initiative and consciously clear your mind of non-productive thoughts. Lingering thoughts that are hanging around creating a depressive atmosphere creates mental anguish.

Clearing Away the Monkey-Brain Chatter

Are you plagued with mental chatter that repeatedly criticizes -- telling you that you are not accomplishing everything that needs to get done? The last thing a person needs is monkey-brain chatter berating you. What a waste of energy!

Our tendency is to pile our plates to excess with responsibilities. Either we unwittingly take on too many duties, or we are not effective time managers. Unfortunately, following glib advice like "just say no when asked to take on additional projects" or "delegate your tasks" isn't always feasible. There are some things we cannot say no to, even though we might like to. And there are certain areas in which we simply are not comfortable allowing another person take over for us -- Hello Control Issues!

Are You Guilty of Wasting Time?

Admittedly, I have been guilty of wasting time. I am still learning about time efficiency. Whenever I am in a state of avoidance or am having difficulty making a decision, I tend to make myself very busy doing other things. This way I can attempt to fool myself into believing that I'm not really avoiding anything, I'm simply too busy to get around to everything. What a load of crap! Can you tell that I'm not very good at convincing myself?

Pesky tasks I have neglected to tend to will continue to haunt me until I settle down and actually get around to doing them. It is usually not until I take the bull by the horns and finish the daunting activity that I realize just how much time and energy I wasted in mental anguish during my avoidance period. Why didn't I just roll-up my sleeves and get to work on that project to begin with? When will I ever learn?

While Avoiding Something, It Is Probably Not Avoiding You

You may have put a particular task on the back-burner, choosing to ignore it for a few days, weeks, or even months. Meanwhile, the uncomfortable "undone-ness" of whatever it is you are avoiding is likely simmering away in the back of your mind making a nuisance of itself. The whole time the stream of hot steam emitting from that stew pot will be blurring or blocking your thought processes. The nagging reminders of unfinished business that clutter our minds is very heavy on the heart and can also effect our overall health negatively.

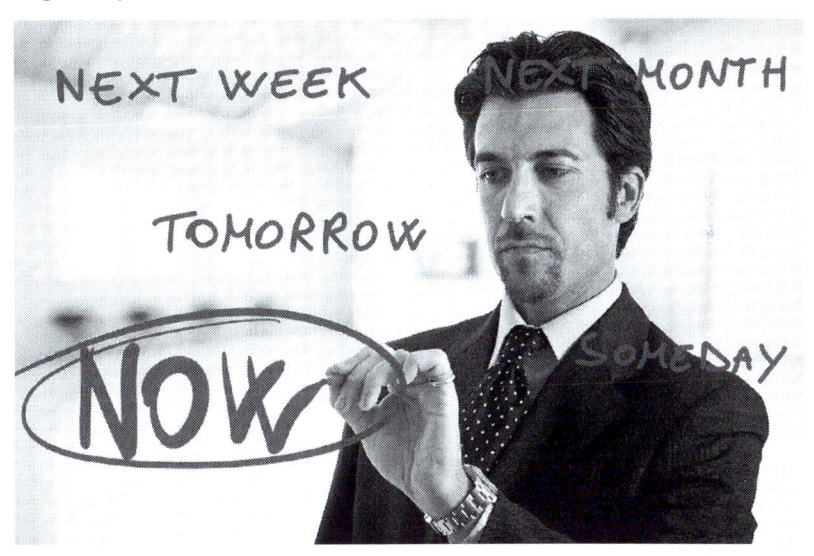

Avoidance, Procrastination, and Indecision Contribute to Mental Anguish

My best advice is to avoid avoidance at all costs. Stop stressing over your indecision, breathe deep into your gut and take a leap of faith. Don't worry that your decisions may turn out less than wonderful. You'll never know for sure until you allow something new or different a chance to evolve anyway.

Take Action and Tackle Those Pesky Tasks

Take action and do whatever it is that you have been intending to do but never get around to it because it isn't the most pleasant task to attend to. You will feel so much better having put it behind you. Completing your tasks will purge those nagging thoughts of unfinished business from your mind. Tackle the pesky tasks one by one. Just Do It! You'll be happier and healthier for it.

11. Balancing and centring

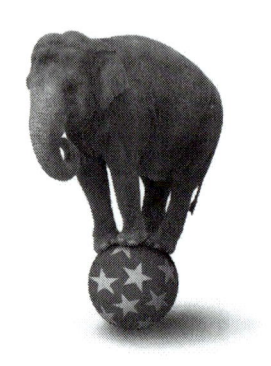

These are some visualizations meant to help you ground and find balance. Because our energies are always in flux it is important to "check in" with our bodies (both physical and energy bodies) routinely to adjust and centre ourselves. If you find yourself stubbing your toes or bumping into things, you are not in balance. If you are experiencing mental confusion or are all over the place emotionally, a centring visualization can help return you to calm and better focus.

12. Let Go and Break Free

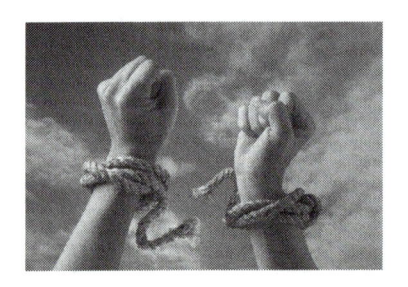

Are you having difficulty walking away from a toxic relationship? Or do you tend to dwell on the past instead of moving forward in your life? Choose images in your visualization sessions which will allow you to break free from problematic people and move past personal regrets. We cannot change the past, but we can create our futures. Begin a new way of living by visualizing it first!

How To Live Your Life Without Regrets

(By Phylameana lila Desy, About.com Guide)

Everyone has made poor choices or done something in their past that could possibly be labelled as "regrettable." But, think about it. The fact that you are now able to look back and realize that a mistake or miss-step occurred means you have learned a valuable lesson. Some of my choices may have landed me in unpleasant circumstances, but experiencing these things certainly built my current character. I wouldn't be where I am today if it weren't for those character-building situations. Mistakes are stepping stones to an evolving life. No need for you to sink into regret or despair -- keep your chin up.

<u>Here's How to do it:</u>

1. <u>Acknowledge a mistake has been made</u> - It is easy to play the blame game, pointing fingers at someone else or circumstances as to why you have stumbled or why your life is difficult. Taking personal ownership that your past actions resulted in bringing about your current reality is the first step to moving past regrets and moving toward a brighter future.

2. <u>Make amends</u> - If your past actions or words have harmed another person an apology may be in order. Or not, apologies can be tricky. Judge for yourself if an apology will help matters or only drudge up old wounds better left alone. But, definitely forgive yourself! Nobody is perfect. We all make mistakes. Continually berating yourself for past actions is self-defeating. Would you kick a dog while it was laying down? Of course not. Please don't do this to yourself. Righting a wrong is not always feasible. If you feel badly about a past action you've taken that cannot be righted, forgive yourself, and let it go.

3. <u>Do-overs</u> - Sometimes feelings of regret arise not from our past actions, but from our non-actions. Have you ever regretted not taking a vacation, staying stuck in a dead-end job, not attending college... or whatever? It may be too late to reverse those decisions, but you still have options. Some colleges offer free classes for seniors. You might not have the time, money, or physical endurance to travel, but you can rent movies or attend travelogue showings about the regions you wish to learn more about. New opportunities are available around every corner if you just open your heart and follow your dreams.

4. Be grateful - The most valuable lessons learned in life often come from the mistakes we make. It may take a walk down a dark alley to see clearly. Embrace your follies, feel gratitude for getting past the worst episodes and eventually finding your way along a less-cluttered path.

5. Be careful not to repeat the same mistake - A skinned-knee teaches a small child not to run so fast. Slow-down. If you are repeatedly faced with similar difficulties over and over again, this is a sure bet that you have not learned the lessons these situations are trying to teach. Opportunity will surface only after you take responsibility for faulty actions taken and change your current and future behaviours accordingly.

6. Be watchful of future knee-jerk reactions - This is probably the toughest step, not reacting negatively to situations or the people who tend to push your buttons. We don't always have control over the things life tosses in front of us, but we do control our reactions. Stay calm. Introduce stress-management into your daily life. Meditation helps clear and focus the mind. Therapeutic play will help balance work-related stresses.

7. Looking deeper inside - Re-evaluate the direction your life is taking. Have you accepted that your past mistakes are just that --- in the past? Focus on today. Become aware of your future goals and desires. Setting clear intentions will help clear the path so that your life progresses with a freer heart and increased happiness. The best is yet to come! Believe it.

Tips:

1. Remember, nobody is perfect. Including yourself!
2. Forgiveness is golden.
3. Live for today. Yesterday was then.

Sources:

http://www.nursingstudentsupport.net/content/SAPDF/SM20.Mental Imagery.pdf

http://akoven.tripod.com/healingwithhypnosis/id8.html

Visualization discovery Tour

By Phylameana lila Desy, About.com Guide

http://healing.about.com/od/visualization/ss/visualization-discovery-tour.htm

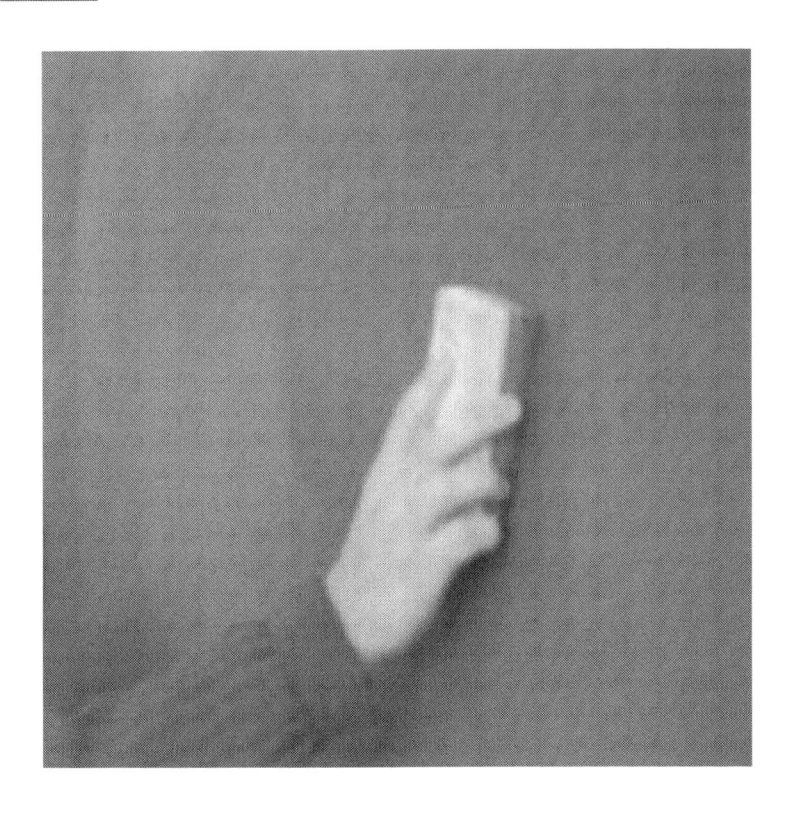

2. When, Why, How Use Mental Imagery?

2.1 Relaxation and Meditation

Use tranquil natural scenes: images that place you in a peaceful, natural environment or images that reflect a relaxed state (Buddha, leaf floating on river, person descending staircase, meditating person)

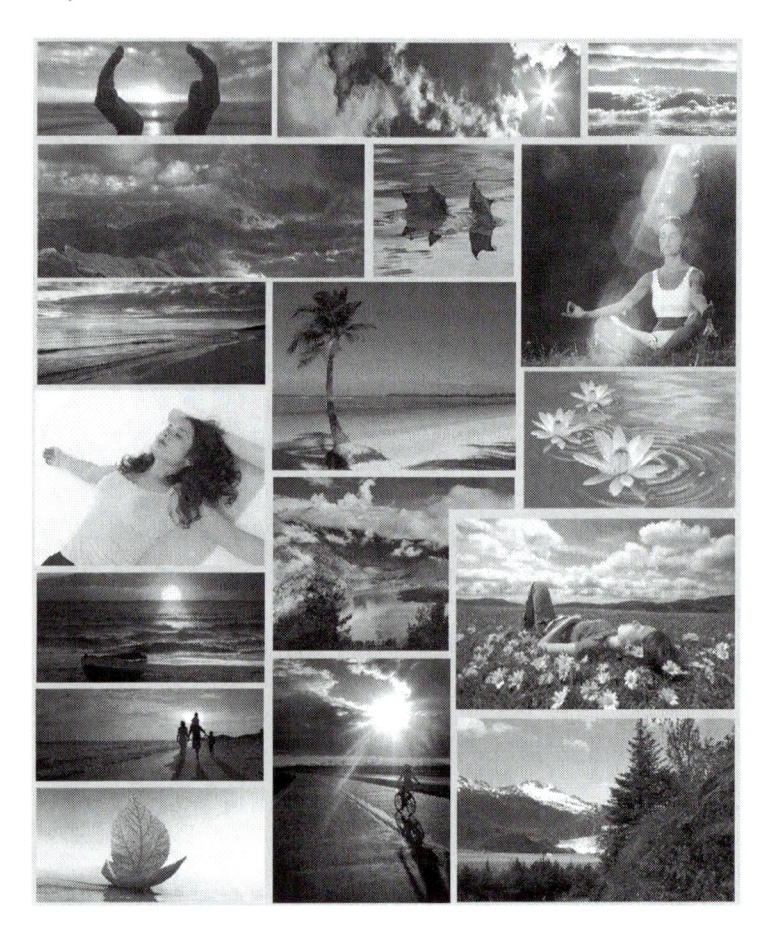

2.2 Building Confidence and Readiness

Seeing yourself perform skills at a high level, the way you want to: confident, accurate, focused, ... is a good way to build confidence and a feeling of readiness prior to a challenging task (public presentation, important meeting, ...) or competition.

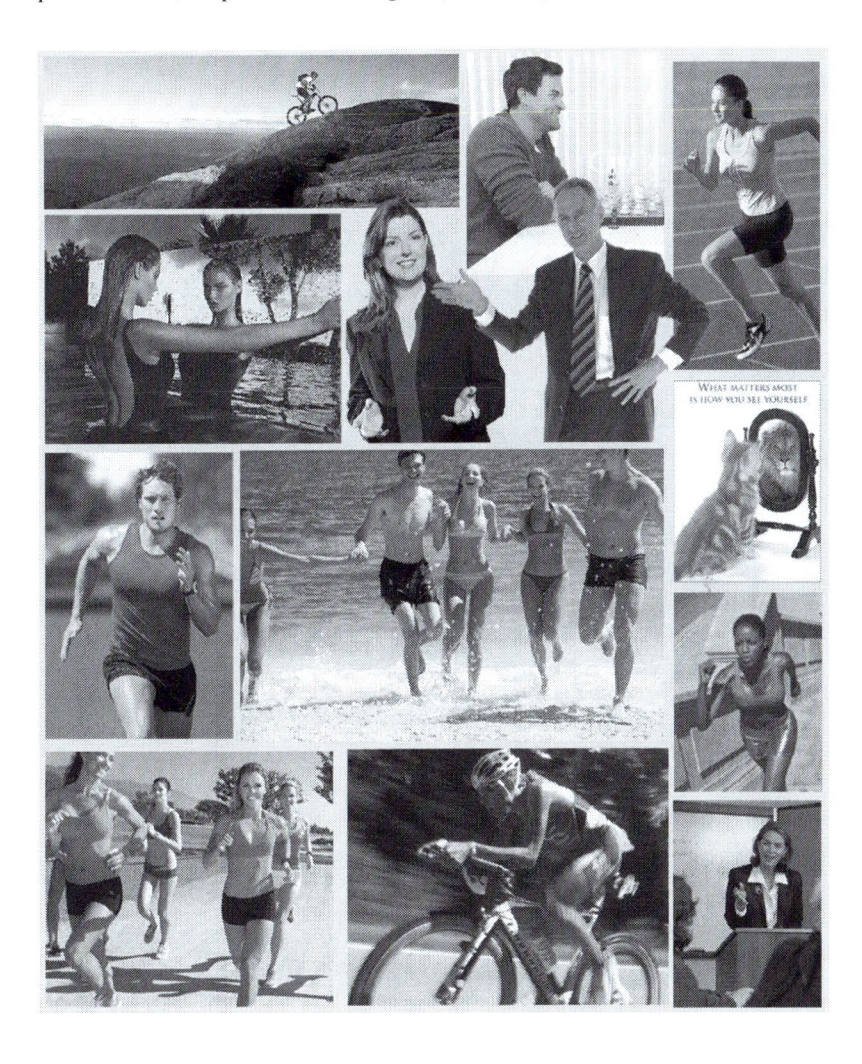

2.3 Preparing Success

Achieving your goals, being successful and being who you want to be and living the life you want, is best visualized by mentally rehearsing the positive outcomes of future actions and events and by picturing the destined future stage.

Envision yourself achieving your goals vividly to remind yourself of your objective and what you need to do to reach it. Many athletes, actors, and singers "see" and "feel" themselves performing a routine, program, or play perfectly before they actually do it.

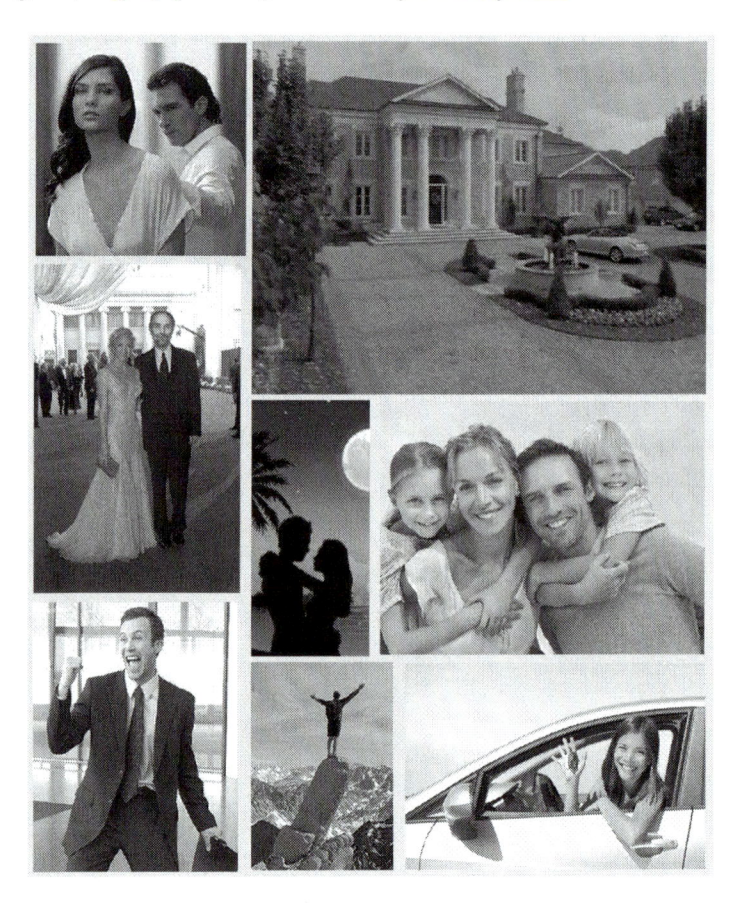

2.4 Familiarizing

Familiarizing or setting the stage for a performance or event.

Mental imagery can be used effectively to familiarize yourself with the surroundings before an event, such as an interview, an important meeting, a sales conversation or negotiation, a public presentation, a competition site, a racetrack, a stage or a difficult play or routine prior to a competition ...

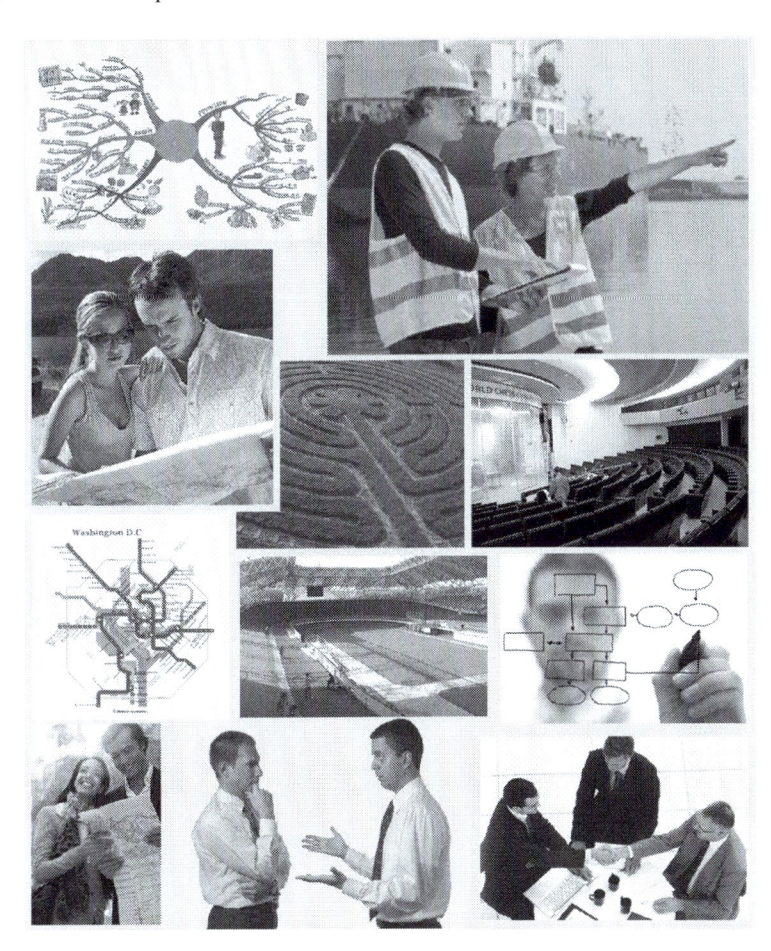

2.5 Doing a run-through.

It can also be used as a cognitive technique to plan strategies, rehearse procedures or game plans, affirm what you want to occur, or as a coping skill strategy to stay calm and composed under pressure. Athletes and performers often do a complete mental run through of the key elements of their routines. This helps them focus, eliminate some pre-performance jitters and be more comfortable. It also serves as a warm-up or mini rehearsal.

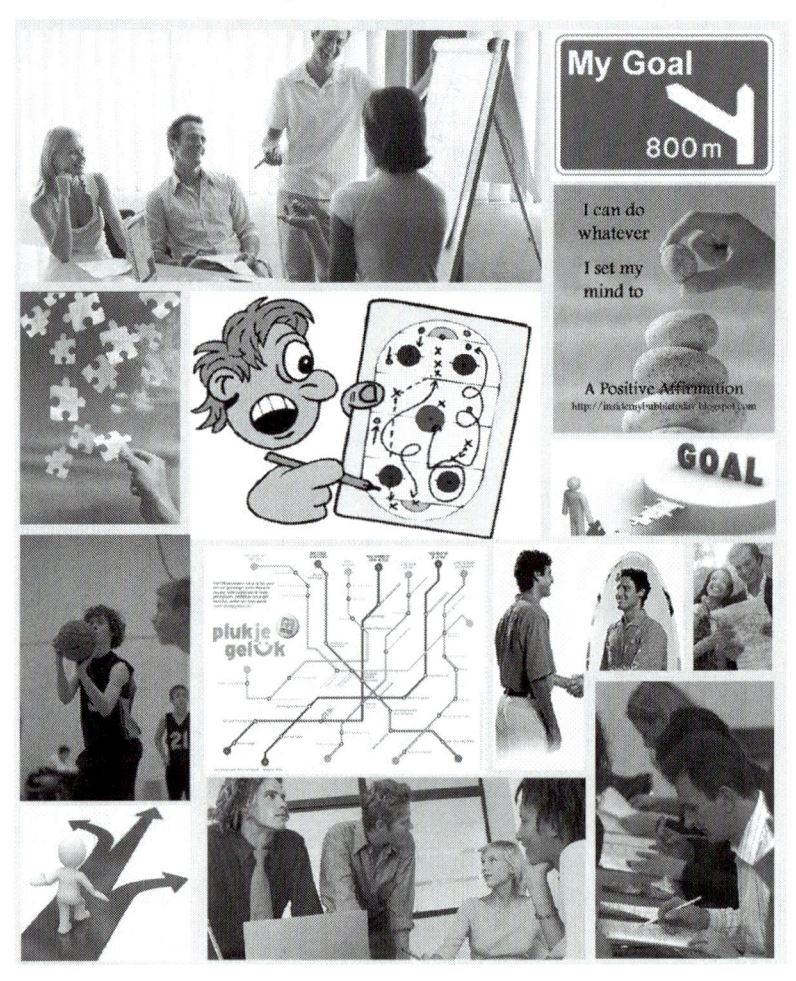

2.6 Healing and Recovery

Internal body images or images of trips inside the body to observe and repair damaged tissue. The most effective images are the ones that have some meaning to you. You may imagine your ailment as an enemy that you attack, or how some external force (nature, God, angel, ...) helps you to push it back. Another way is to imagine how your life will be again after you conquered the sickness.

For instance, when healing tumours, people might imagine that their healthy cells are plump, juicy berries, while their cancerous cells are dried, shrivelled pieces of fruit. They might picture their immune system as birds that fly in and pick up and carry away the raisin-like cancer cells, while the rest of the cells flourish. Another common image is that the immune system cells are like silver bullets coming in and annihilating the tumour cells.

Other experts recommend actually personifying your condition and "reasoning" with it. This way you also have a chance to learn from your condition. If you're plagued by headaches, for example, you might imagine your headache as a gremlin tightening a vice across your temples. Ask the gremlin why he's there and what you Ask the gremlin why he's there and what you can do to make him loosen his grip. He might "tell" you that you have had too little sleep, too much junk food, or not enough rest and time away from work. Take his advice, and there is a good chance your headaches will subside, experts say.

Case example 1:

I sit in a quiet place (if at all possible). I close my eyes gently and take a few deep breaths. During this time, my mind travels to the spleen and watches as red blood cells (rbcs) come out to travel around the body. They travel to the heart and to the lungs and I watch as they pick up oxygen and return to the heart to be sent to all parts of the body. At this time, the rbcs have also picked up glucose and there are white blood cells and antibodies travelling with them. I view them as they descend through the network of arteries, arterioles, and capillaries and then, they are at the sites that need healing. I like to visualize the right and left sides separately, but if I am tired and start fighting sleep, then I pull my perspective back and watch both sides at the same time. I see the rbcs leaving oxygen and glucose at the base of the lesions. I see the antibodies surrounding the areas to prevent infection and I see the wbcs backing up the antibodies.

I then pull my perspective back and gently stroke each arm separately and visualize more blood going to the areas to help them heal. The last thing I do is to take several deep breaths and tell my body that I do not want it to show me evidence of my anger, frustration, or stress. I tell it that there is no need for my body to hurt itself. Then I take three long breaths out and with each exhale I say (imaginally): "With this breath, I breathe out all of my anger, with this breath, I breathe out all of my stress, with this breath I breath out all my frustration."

Case example 2

Sandra has been asthmatic since childhood. Despite using a variety of approaches, she has always felt enslaved to her disease. She has tried both ignoring her condition and catering to it. Though everything seems to help for a time, nothing gives her the release she seeks. Feeling drained and confused, she seeks out a clinician trained in the use of mental imagery as a treatment of last resort.

The therapist asks Sandra to close her eyes, turns her senses inward, and does some reverse breathing (exhaling first though her mouth, then inhaling through her nose). With this simple preparation, Sandra enters the world of her imagination where anything is possible – for here there are no rules, no diagnoses or prognoses, in fact, no limitations of any kind. Using an imagery exercise called "Liberation From Slavery," Sandra sees and feels herself chained to her illness which appears to her as a large beast pressing her down, its foot planted firmly on her chest. Uncomfortable as this image may be, once she sees it she has the opportunity to acknowledge it (in effect to experience it), and to make a change. Using her imagination, she finds a key that unlocks the chains, breaks free of the beast, and releases herself from its power. Suddenly, the beast begins shrinking, while Sandra grows taller. As the chains fall away, the restriction and heaviness in her chest diminish. She feels lighter, her breathing becomes easier, and the sense of fear and powerlessness she had been feeling is replaced by hope and clarity.

When the imagery exercise is completed, the clinician as the guide, instructs her to breathe out and open her eyes. At this time, the therapist asks Sandra how she feels, and asks Sandra to describe her experience from the exercise in the present tense. She is encouraged to try this exercise (the prescribed dose), every day for at least seven days, up to 21 days, and to record her experiences (including night dreams) until her next appointment.

The benefits Sandra derives from doing this exercise are far reaching and immediate. Her imagery acts as a mirror that reveals her from the inside out. Instantaneously, from the imagery exercise she has learned truths about herself that until now she has overlooked, even denied. Indeed, she is stronger, "taller," more powerful than she ever suspected. By freeing herself from the chains (which she sensed were her beliefs and fears about her illness), she becomes bigger than this disease, something she had always felt was all powerful, too much for her to handle. In changing the image, which she does by using the key to release herself, she has affected her beliefs, thoughts, and feelings in a positive, and liberating way. In doing this, she has gone beyond ordinary thinking where such things are "impossible," and has become her own authority, the one who is ultimately in control of her choices in life (Shafer & Greenfield, 2002).

Source:

http://healing.about.com/od/visualization/a/imagery_shafer.htm
Imagine Yourself Well
By Kathryn C. Shafer, Ph.D.

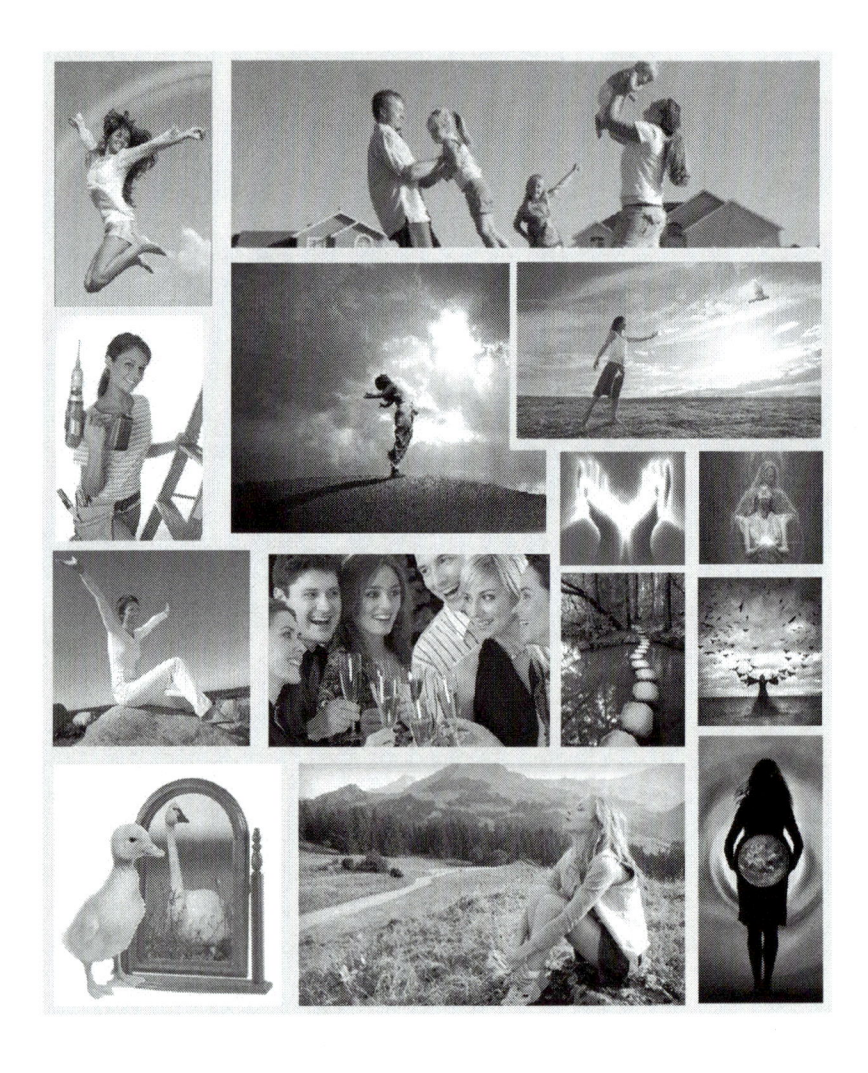

2.7 Behaviour Change

Go for images that allow you to see and feel yourself act in the new way and reap the advantages of the change. You could promote a different, more health-conscious behaviour this way, a new leaderships-style, a new way of approaching challenges and problems, a life without cigarettes and alcohol, ...

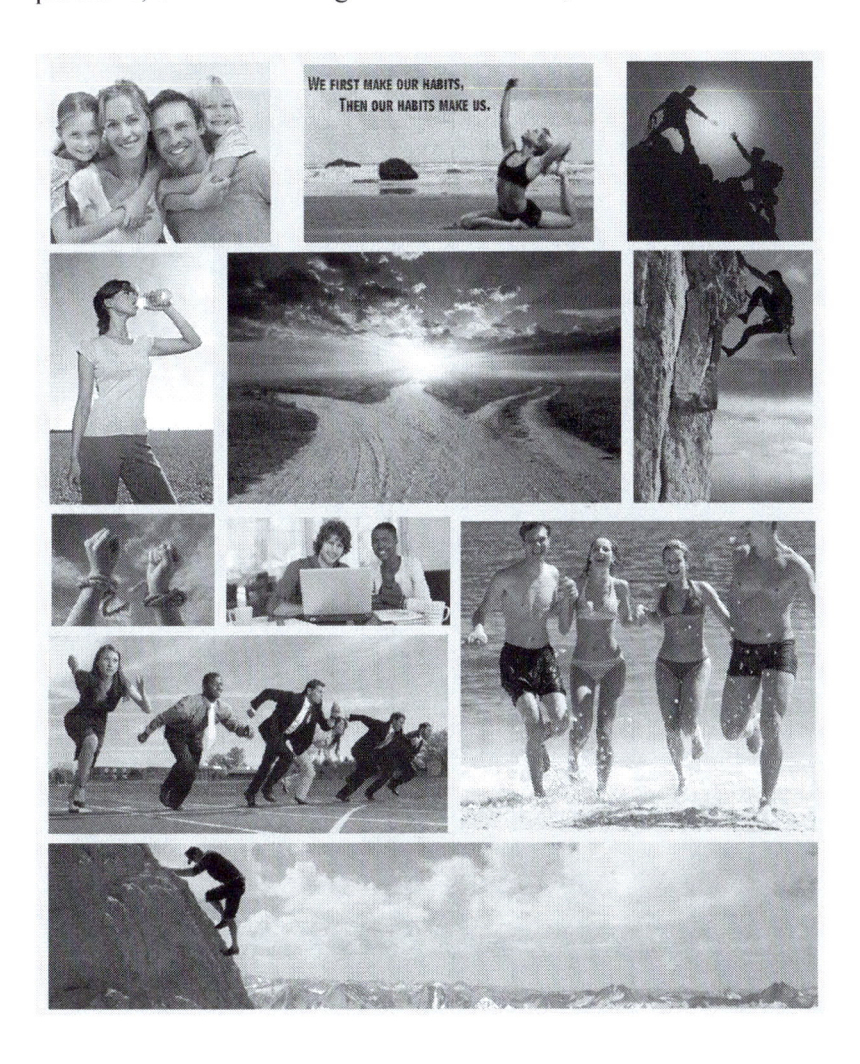

You can use visualization for anything and everything that you want to prepare for in advance. It helps you be more comfortable and perform at a higher level no matter what. It's a great way to rehearse and prepare for any kind of event or situation.

Source: http://www.mascsa-psu.edu/dave/Visualization-handout.pdf

By David Yukeson, Ph.D. Penn State University.

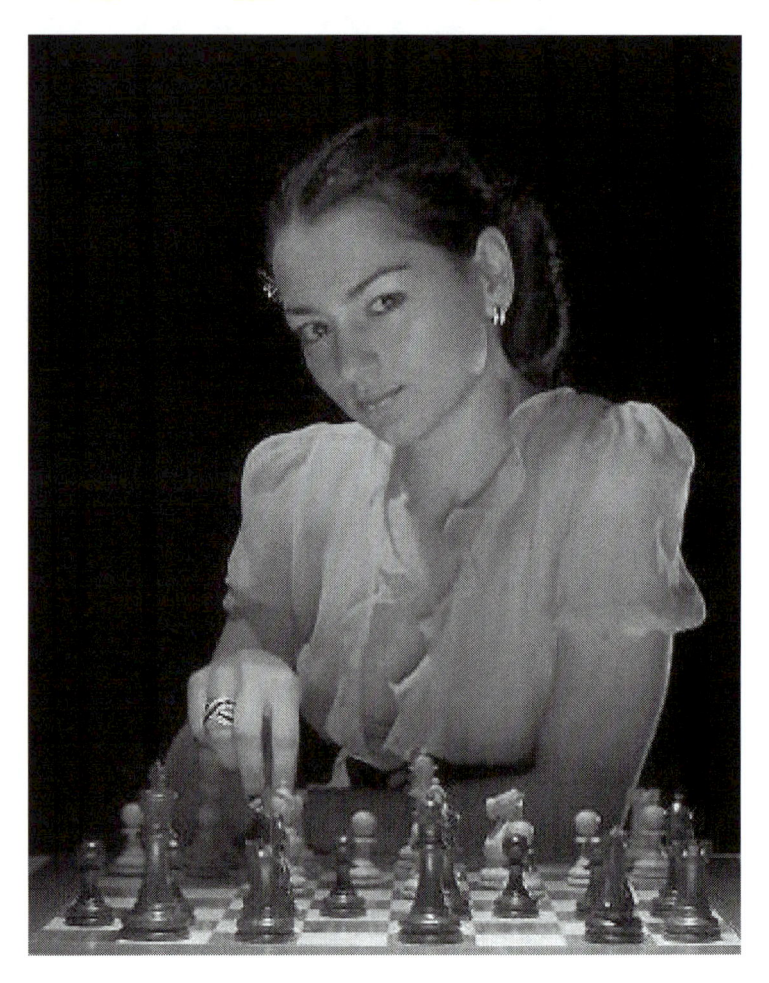

3. How To Develop Imagery Skills?

The aim of this page is to help you develop your imagery (visualization) skills. We will look at the elements of imagery development and the creation of scripts to help in developing your imagery skills.

3.1 Imagery Categories

The five main categories of imagery have been identified as follows:

1. Motivational-specific (MS)

This involves seeing yourself winning an event, receiving a trophy or medal and being congratulated by other athletes. MS imagery may boost motivation and effort during training and facilitate goal-setting, but is unlikely on its own to lead directly to performance benefits

2. Motivational general-mastery (MG-M)

This is based on seeing yourself coping in difficult circumstances and mastering challenging situations. It might include maintaining a positive focus while behind, and then coming back to win. MG-M imagery appears to be important in developing expectations of success and self-confidence

3. Motivational general-arousal (MG-A)

This is imagery that reflects feelings of relaxation, stress, anxiety or arousal in relation to sports competitions. There is good evidence to suggest that MG-A imagery can influence heart rate - one index of arousal - and can be employed as a 'psych-up' strategy

4. Cognitive specific (CS)

This involves seeing yourself perform specific skills, such as a tennis serve, golf putt or triple-toe-loop in figure skating. If learning and performance are the desired outcomes, evidence suggests that CS imagery will be the most effective choice

5. Cognitive general (CG)

This involves images of strategy and game plans related to a competitive event. Examples could include employing a serve-and-volley strategy in tennis or a quick-break play in basketball.

3.2 Where Do I Start?

To be effective, like any skill, imagery needs to be developed and practiced regularly. There are four elements to mental imagery: Relaxation, Realism, Regularity and Reinforcement (the 4Rs)

1. Relaxation

Having a relaxed mind and body so you can become involved in the imagery exercises, feel your body moving and experience any emotions generated. It may help to use a relaxation technique prior to imagery training.

2. Realism

Create imagery so realistic you believe you are actually executing the skill. In order to obtain the most realistic imagery possible, you must incorporate clarity, vividness, emotion, control and a positive outcome into your imagery:

- Clarity - Make the images as vivid as possible, include color
- Vividness - Incorporate as many of your senses as possible into your imagery so the scene is as clear and realistic as real life itself

- Emotion - Try to include emotional feelings in your images. Refresh your memory constantly by emphasizing specific sensory awareness (e.g. smells, the wind) during training
- Control - Break down the image into small components and visualize those components. (Sprinting - consider the action of the arms, legs, trunk, head, feet, hands, breathing etc.)
- Positive outcome - This is essential, "you only achieve what you believe"

3. Regularity

Spending between 3 and 5 minutes on imagery seems to be most effective. It should be included in training and time outside of training should be spent on imagery. (10-15 minutes a day)

4. Reinforcement

The writing of imagery scripts will help you plan the content and timing of your imagery training.

3.3 Creating a Script

1. Basic picture

Outline the basic content of the act or situation to be imagined - write it in the first person (I). To describe a skill execution, make sure you include all components of the skill to be imagined or behaviours to be emphasised, especially if it is a complex skill. If you are describing the events in a sport situation, include all actions that occur in the event and the correct sequencing of all the actions.

2. Add details

Add the sensory stimuli - the descriptors (adjectives) that add colour, detail (e.g. context, weather) and movement qualities (e.g. speed of movement) to the original script components or events.

Add the movement or kinaesthetic feelings, physiological or body responses, and the emotional responses. The words that are added are action words such as verbs and adverbs that clearly describe the quality of actions or emotions.

3. Refine the script

Read it to yourself and try to imagine the event in all its sensory, action and emotional detail. Do you feel as if you are actually executing the skill or experiencing the event? If not, re-examine the descriptors and action words to see if they accurately reflect the sensations associated with this action.

4. Tape it

When you have a suitable script then record it on to audiotape and you can then use it as a prompt for your imagery training.

Example - Tennis Serve

- Basic Story - Components:
- Preparation,
- Ball toss,
- Impact,
- Recovery,
- Ball flight and
- landing in service box

5. Add more details

See the racket in the hand, the bright yellow ball rebounding against the green court as you bounce it in preparation, see the position of the opponent, look at the point on the court where you will direct the serve.

- feeling the relaxed shoulders and hands
- feeling the racket grip in the hand

- seeing the bright yellow ball nestled on the fingers in the hand
- feeling the smooth release of the ball at the arm's full stretch
- feeling the body weight shift, the knees bend
- feeling the body rising upward as the knees extend
- feeling the power in the body
- feeling the racket head accelerate
- feeling the wrist snap and the sound of the racket making contact with the hall
- watching the ball swerve and land in the centre corner of the green service box and kick away for a clean ace
- feeling the exhilaration and pleasure

6. Refine the script some more

Rewrite the script until when you read it, you feel as if you are executing the serve.

3.4 FITT

In designing your imagery program, apply the FITT principals, as we do with physical training

- **F is for Frequency** - Aim to incorporate imagery into every day of your training schedule. For busy people, just before you sleep could be a good time, and it helps if you are in a relaxed and tranquil state

- **I is for Intensity** - Try to create an all-sensory experience that is as vivid and clear as possible. Initially, practicing in a quiet environment can help to minimize distractions and facilitate clear images

- **T is for Time** - Imagery should make big demands on your attention, so short (5-10 minutes) frequent quality sessions are preferable to long ones

- **T is for Type** - Remember to decide on your desired outcome and select the type of imagery to match it.

How to Visualize What you want:

1. Go somewhere quiet and private where you won't be disturbed. Close your eyes and think of the goal, mood, new behaviour or skill, you want to acquire.
2. Take several deep breaths and relax.
3. Visualize the object or situation you desire in your mind as clearly and with as much detail as you can.
4. Add emotion, feeling, and your senses to your vision.
5. Practice it at least twice a day for about 10 minutes each time.
6. Persevere until you succeed.
7. Maintain positive thoughts and a good attitude throughout.

The Benefits of Visualization

- Helps you focus better in order to achieve your goals
- Inspires and motivates you.
- Helps you improve in a sport or skill.
- Can be used to rehearse and then acquire new, positive behaviors.
- Can boost your mood by using positive, pleasant imagery to alter negative emotions.
- Helps build self-confidence.

3.5 Practical Examples

3.5.1 How To Visualize Confidence

All of us would like more confidence. Whether you need more body confidence, confidence in interviews, confidence in relationships, or career confidence, I'm sure there's an area of your life that could do with a confidence boost.

But what if you could use the power of visualization and mental imagery to enable your brain to allow you to be confident in that situation?

Studies in mental imagery have shown that the brain cannot distinguish from a real or an imaginary picture. The same chemicals release and the same electrical activity displays in the brain whether we are visualizing something or actually doing it.

A repeated thought, or feeling, can actually become a belief over time. Have you ever been constantly thinking about a particular outcome in a positive sense that you actually felt good about it?

What I mean is that you can actually train your mind to be confident.

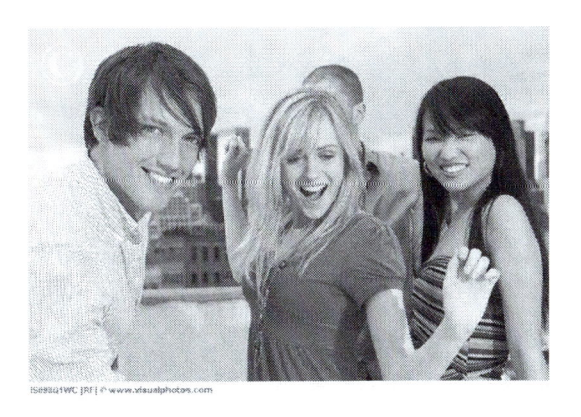

It's similar to the well known conditioning experiment, Pavlov's dogs, whereby every time they fed the dogs, the researchers rang a bell at the same time. After repeated times of doing this, just ringing the bell would make the dogs salivate. It was an unconscious response to something that had been neurologically linked in their mindset- the association between food and the bell.

Imagine if you could make similar connections between confidence and getting that job for example, or every time you looked at your body you automatically feel good.

Of course, like in the experiment this takes a bit of time, but the great thing is you will feel in control of your confidence, rather than the other way around.

Here's 5 Ways to Visualize Yourself Confident:

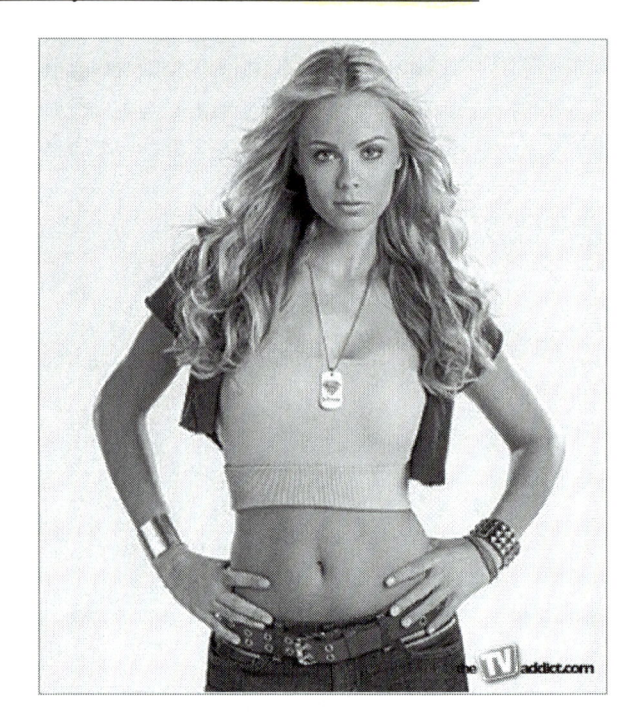

1. Think of a time you were really, really confident. Imagine every detail, as if you were looking through your own eyes. See, hear and feel those great feelings. Squeeze your index finger and thumb together whilst doing this (you may have heard of this technique, which is called anchoring). After several times of doing this just squeezing your index finger and thumb alone should produce some positive and confident feelings. Use this 'anchor' when you are thinking about or in the situation you'd like to have more confidence in.

2. Visual Mental Rehearsal: Think of a specific situation in relation to your confidence. For example, if you'd like more confidence in a social situation, imagine yourself there. See it as if it was a movie, seeing yourself laughing and talking easily and effortlessly with others. Visualize this as often as you can, and you can even listen to some upbeat music so you feel good when you're imagining.

3. Get into the physiology of confidence: Think of someone you know who is really confident. Vividly imagine how their posture looks, how they carry themselves, how they walk and talk, how loud they speak, how they sit, how they greet people. Now, get yourself into consciously training your body to act in the same way. Keep a mental check on yourself and change your posture, your tone of voice, your body language. Just simple changes can give you an instant confidence boost anywhere.

4. Eliminate self doubt through autosuggestion. You know how powerful adverts are? That's because they deliver a repeated message which sinks into our unconscious mind. You can create messages to yourself and continually reaffirm them when visualizing. It can be something as simple as ' I conduct my presentation with ease and confidence'. You can say the phrase out loud or imagine that you saying it to themselves and see yourself feeling good.

5. Increase self esteem by focusing on appreciation. People who have higher self esteem and self-worth usually have higher levels of confidence, so when you visualize yourself in that situation, focus on that you as a friend, someone you would like to help and encourage. Allow that you to begin to appreciate all of the amazing qualities of you. For example, if you would like more dating confidence, imagine seeing yourself through the eyes of someone who loves you and admires you. Focus on all of your strengths and imagine what your future partner may appreciate and love about you.

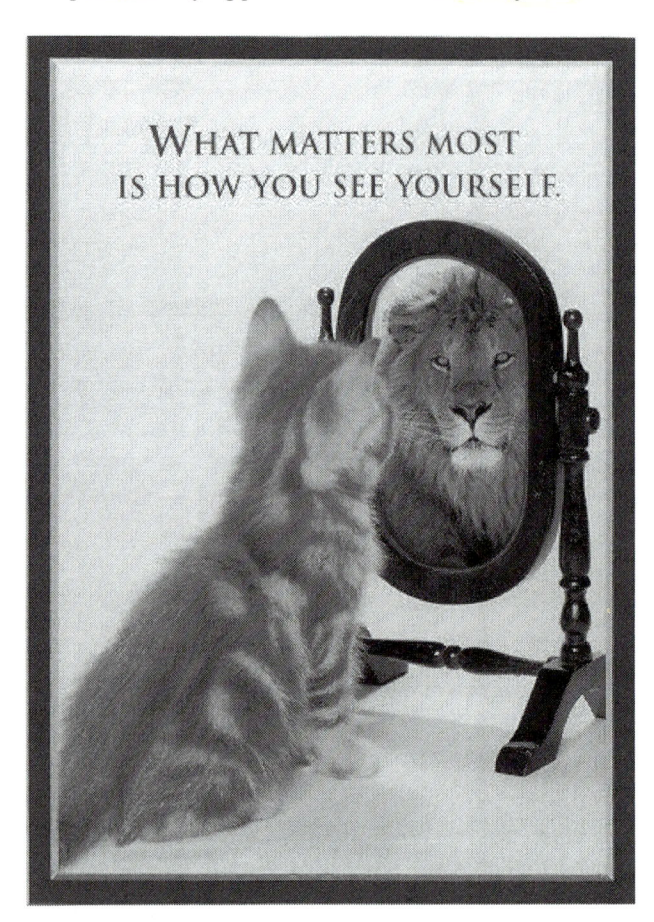

WHAT MATTERS MOST IS HOW YOU SEE YOURSELF.

3.5.2 Use Mental Imagery for Achieving Success

1. Image Resource and Relaxation

We shall show you how to create your image resource and how to use it for relaxing but before going any further, you have to find out your preferred sensory method.

1.1 Discover your best sensory method

Anyone has a preferred method of perception: people are indeed above all sensitive:

either to what they see (visual)
or to what they hear (auditory)
or what they feel or touch.

To determine your preferred method of perception, you will make the following exercise.

Firstly, here is a list of words. Ask someone to read them to you while you are doing the exercise.

A dance	A kitchen	Tulips
A street	A valley	Courage
An apple	A lake	Thunder
An ink pot	A forest	A castle
Wine	A T-shirt	Jazz
Freedom	A river	A meeting

| An office | Money | A leather chair |

As soon as you hear the word, tick straight away the column that seems to best correspond to what comes immediately into your mind:

If an image appears, if you see something in your mind, tick the column V. If you hear a sound or if you repeat the word in your mind, tick A. If you feel a physical sensation or find a taste or smell, tick G.

V	A	G
*	*	*
*	*	
*	*	
*		

Look at the column that is ticked the most. This is your preferred sensory method. Also observe the one that you have only ticked rarely. This is without doubt the sensory method that you use the least. Obviously in the above example, the man who has ticked is a "visual" and secondary an "auditory".

This knowledge of your best sensory method will help you for building your image resource.

1.2 Choose your image resource

Definition: The image resource is a mental image that is to say an image that you see in your mind when your eyes are closed.

MENTAL IMAGERY

DRAWING 1

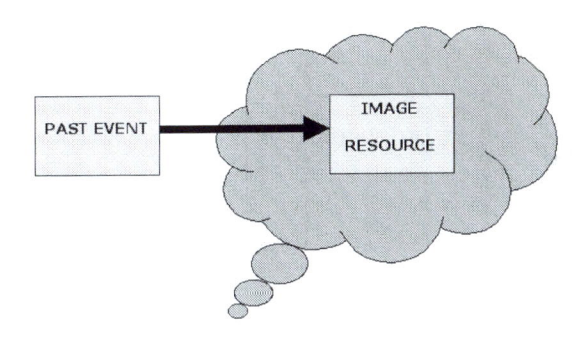

This image resource is the memory of a pleasant situation that you have really experienced in the past.

With this banal memory, you have a work to do for transforming it in a strong mental image which is able to make you relive the feelings that you had experienced in the past.

For example, when you have had a painful experience and when you remember it, you feel again, in a weaker way, the feelings that you had already experienced :you shudder again retrospectively, you go pale.

On the contrary, thanks to your image resource, you should remember your past pleasant feelings and try to live them again as intensely as possible. I mean that your first task is to choose among the flow of your memories, one very pleasant which can fill up some characteristics:

- Your image resource must be a very pleasant image.
- Your image resource must be a very quiet image. Consequently, avoid very moving images such as a dance party or a meeting. A situation where you are alone and at rest must be favoured.

Down to earth advice

Many persons choose the memory of a river as image resource. It could be a good choice because it gives a feeling of quietness. Mountains and green meadows could be also very effective.

You must have a strong feeling of identity with your image resource. For this reason, it's always better to choose it in an environment where you have lived for a long time.

Once your image has been chosen, try to adapt it to your best sensory method. If you are:

o more visual: increase the number of colors
o more auditory: plan for sounds, voices and pleasant melodies that you imagine hearing when looking at the mind-image
o more G: see yourself in your mental image touching things, shaking hands and so on. Imagine smell and perfume and try to live it.

You will use your image resource in many situations and first for relaxing.

1.3 Relaxation techniques

You need to learn how to relax because relaxation is the first step of many process in mental imagery and visioning. We shall give you here our personal method that we experience everyday. Its main advantage is to be easy to use with fast results.

Your image resource is the first thing that you need when you are going to relax. Then you have to choose a quiet place for example your bedroom. Make sure there is no noise to interrupt your relaxation. Remain in half-darkness. Lie down if you are in your bedroom or sit in a position that makes it easy to relax if you are in an office.

When you are in this situation begin to relax:

FIRST SEQUENCE

Close your eyes. Breathe as slowly and as regularly as possible. Say the formula: I am perfectly calm

Imagine your image resource as we have defined it before: For example, a river that flows in the countryside. Mentally develop this image: Look at this image from all sides and try to relive your feelings. It must occupy your whole mind so as not to leave any room for other sensations or ideas.

SECOND SEQUENCE.

Say the following phrases with your inner voice: My left arm is heavy, my two arms are heavy, my legs are heavy, my entire body is heavy.

You should have a vision of your body sinking, disappearing. The aim of this exercise is to make all bodily sensations fade away as much as possible.

THIRD SEQUENCE

Now let's your image resource disappearing. You should be in a pre-sleep condition. Bodily feeling is reduced to its simplest expression. You think of nothing. Your mind is empty.

DRAWING 2 ILLUSTRATES THE RELAXATION PROCESS:

DRAWING 2

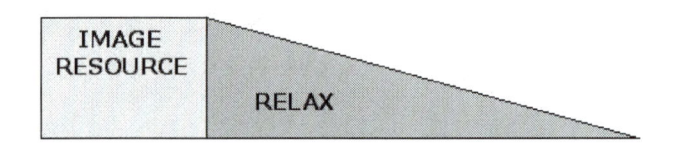

```
| IMAGE    |
| RESOURCE |
|          RELAX          |
```

As you can see, it's look quite easy. In fact you will need to train: Practice this exercise, several times a day. When you have mastered it, you will be able to reach this relaxed state almost instantaneously: Count in your head from 10 to 1.

10 — 9 — 8 — 7 :   carrying out the 1st sequence
6 — 5 — 4 — 3 :   carrying out the second sequence
2 - 1 :   carrying out the 3rd sequence.

By slowly pronouncing 10 — 9 — 8 — 7 up to 1, you will attain the required state of relaxation. Count one month of exercise to reach this automatic mastery.

2. Cleaning the Subconscious

Right now, you have to use your image resource and the relaxation techniques for cleaning your subconscious from all the negative beliefs which are coming from your past.

2. Analysing reality:

2.1 Autobiography.

What do you do when you start a new day? You shower and you wash your body. Now, you are starting a new life: You have to clean your reality. Reality is made up of two things: Your past and your present condition

Your present condition is influenced by your past. As the past no longer exists, it is above all your memories that explain your current state. You are going therefore to examine your past or more precisely the memories and beliefs that you have of it.

Take a pen and paper and write down your life from the beginning. Write down your life chronologically, breaking it down into distinct periods: Childhood, learning period, studies, first job etc. Analyze each period and look for:

- What you wanted at the time
- What was your most outstanding feeling

For example, look at the following imaginary autobiography of a young man that we shall call John:

1970-1975: I don't remember much of my early childhood. I had 2 brothers and 3 sisters. My mother was very busy. My father came home late and beat us. My little brother was very funny. We had good times together. I don't have good memories of this period because of my father.

1975-1987: I started primary school. I learned to read, write and count quickly. My teacher was very nice. Later, I wanted to be a building engineer. Overall, I have good memories of school.

1987-1993: I went to high school. I had great difficulty with literature. In 1990, I went to a vocational to become an accountant.

I had no friends and the other students who were often older than me mocked me. I have very bad memories of this period.

1993-2000: I did my military service in the Navy. I liked the open-air life and the sports a lot. After military service, I found a job as a clerk in an insurance company. I don't earn much.. I don't go out much, I have few friends and I don't have much fun.

2.2 Make a table to use this analysis:

Periods	Would you like to relive this period	Why?
70 — 75	NO	
75 — 87	YES	
87 — 93	NO	
93-2000	YES IN NAVY AND NO AFTER	

Analyze carefully the answers to these questions and look for the true reason. In the periods that you do not like, carefully isolate the past experiences and feelings which were particularly unpleasant. Above all, don't hide anything. As with a psy, recall the shameful events. Tell the truth and the truth will free you. Make a list of these events and prepare you to neutralize them.

2.3 Use image resource: Association-Dissociation

It's a well known fact that our present behaviour is often linked to negative experiences in your past. You have written your autobiography and carefully isolated the unpleasant events. Now, you will neutralize these negative experiences.

Just as you wipe data from your computer's hard disk, removing unnecessary programs, you should wipe your subconscious, removing all the memories of negative experiences.

The first step is to relax. Consequently, do the three sequence of the former exercise. When you are fully relaxed, you imagine a mental screen just like a television screen.

Imagine that you Turn on your screen just like a television and relive the negative experience. Vision the image of the experience and relive your painful feelings (humiliation, shame, rage). In this state, you are fully associated to this negative past experience.

Now, disassociate yourself: Put yourself in the position of an independent observer of the previous image. Watch yourself act as if you were someone else. It is no longer you on the screen, it is your double! You are just a spectator of what you were doing. Let this dissociated image takes over your mental screen.

DRAWING 3

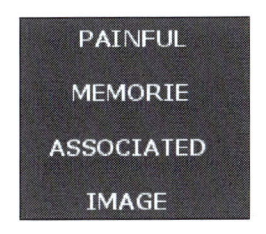

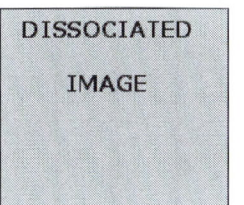

PAINFUL MEMORIE ASSOCIATED IMAGE	DISSOCIATED IMAGE

The black square shows the negative experience when you are reliving it. It's quite painful. The gray square shows the same experience when you have dissociated from it.

On this mental screen, imagine a small square where you look at and relive your image resource (the flowing river for example). Relive it to the maximum leaving the rest of the screen occupied by the negative experience from which your were dissociated.

Enlarge the square of your image resource on the mental screen so that the image of the unpleasant experience disappears completely. It will disappear quickly because you are now fully associated with your image resource.

DRAWING 4

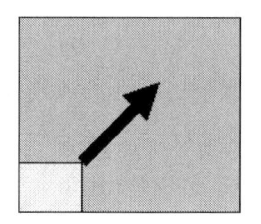

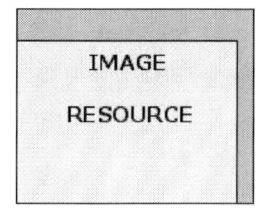

IMAGE RESOURCE

On the drawing, the little blue square represents your image resource which is then enlarged to occupy your entire screen.

Proceed like that for all the unpleasant events you have listed. By the end, you will completely clean up your past and your subconscious.

Be very careful with the people that were witnesses to your negative experiences. Each time you meet them, you can expect they will remind you of those negative periods: "Do you remember when you made us laugh with your exam? and so on"

The cleaning work will be called into question each time you meet them. With a simple look, they will reinstall all your negative beliefs. Only one solution : Don't see them any more, avoid them, eliminate all witnesses to your past lack of success.

2.4 Surf on Troubles

Whatever you do, you will come across difficult experiences in your current situation. For example, you know that an event will go badly. For avoiding to built up a new negative experience, you will cross the event as if you were outside it, as if you were not concerned.

For this purpose, you will use the anchoring method that relies on using a stimulation (image or gesture) that automatically provokes an internal representation. For example: Seeing a blackboard (visual anchor) inspires classroom memories. Listening to a song inspires memories of a party (auditory anchoring).

The stimulation may be visual : remove your glasses, auditory : listen to a song, kinaesthetic: Tighten your fists. Its aim is to produce when needed the desired emotional state to deal with a given situation.

For implementing an anchoring, use the following technique:

As soon as you have reached the relaxation stage, keep it and associate a simple movement with your image resource, like for example, clenching the fist. Restart the operation as often as possible to create a conditioned reflex.

Subsequently, each time that you need your image resource, clench your fist. This gesture will help you to find it, without having to put yourself in a relaxed state.

When you are confronting a painful event, clench your fist, call your image resource. Focus on your image resource and cross the event as though it did not concern you. When the event is finished, all that will remain is a dissociated image and not an associated one that would harm your subconscious.

You have not to be involved in unpleasant events. With your image resource, you surf on the events that you do not like!

2.5 Now rewrite your life!

When you have cleaned your past, you can re-write your personal history eliminating all the negative periods and experiences. This is the history with which you will confront immediate reality. Rather than pulling yourself back, this history will push you forward.

Clean the past and the John's history becomes:

1970-2000: I had some good times with my younger brother. I learned quickly and easily at primary school. The Navy gave me a lot of self-confidence. I am very good at sports and open-air life. I am working for a short period in a financial office. I am making the most of this job to learn some tips useful for starting a biz: I want in the next future to create my own sports business. I am confident: I will enjoy a success story!

Obviously, John must eliminate his bad witnesses: He must not see any more his father, his elder sister who complained all the time or his colleagues at the vocational school. On the contrary, he must get in touch with his brother, his teacher and colleagues of Navy.

Positive beliefs make you see reality as a spring to success. Right now, you are free to choose your vision and that vision will transport you in a successful world.

2.6 External readings

Go to http://mentalhelp.net . Click on "psychological self help". There is a complementary reading about what you have just learnt. You can also click on "tests" to realize some psychological tests.

2.7 Lesson summary

The knowledge of your best sensory method will help you for building your image resource: Your image resource is a mental image that is to say an image that you see in your mind when your eyes are closed.

This image resource is the memory of a pleasant situation that you have really experienced in the past.

You will use your image resource in many situations and first for relaxing and for cleaning your subconscious from all the negative beliefs which are coming from your past.

Once, you have cleaned your past, you can re-write your personal history eliminating all the negative periods and experiences. Rather than pulling yourself back, this history will push you forward.

2.8 Do It Yourself Now:

You have a lot of things to do:

1. First, you must write your autobiography. We recommend you to reread your bio the day after a good night. Do the job in one shot during a week-end when you are not disturbed. Look at your old photos. They could ease the remembrance process. Count about 5 hours of full work for this task

2. Make the exercise about the sensory preference and then, choose your image resource. In writing your bio, you have certainly isolated an event that you would like to relive. Describe completely your image resource. If possible, paint it. Count at least 5 hours for the choice of your image resource.

3. Then, begin the relaxation exercises as described above: Each day, practice 4 exercises during 15 days. As each exercise could last 15

minutes, it means that you have to plan 15 hours of training within these two weeks. Do not go to the visioning module as long as you are not able to relax in the way we have explained

4. Mastering your image resource, you have to eliminate the negative experiences. You should need about five days for eliminating them but the duration depends on your life. In the same way, use the anchoring process and also begin to avoid people bearing negative influence. Count about 8 hours to perform the Tasks.

5. Finally, rewrite your life (Count only 2 hours as you mainly write an abstract)

It means that all these tasks need about 35 hours within a month. When all these tasks have be done, you can enter in the visioning course.

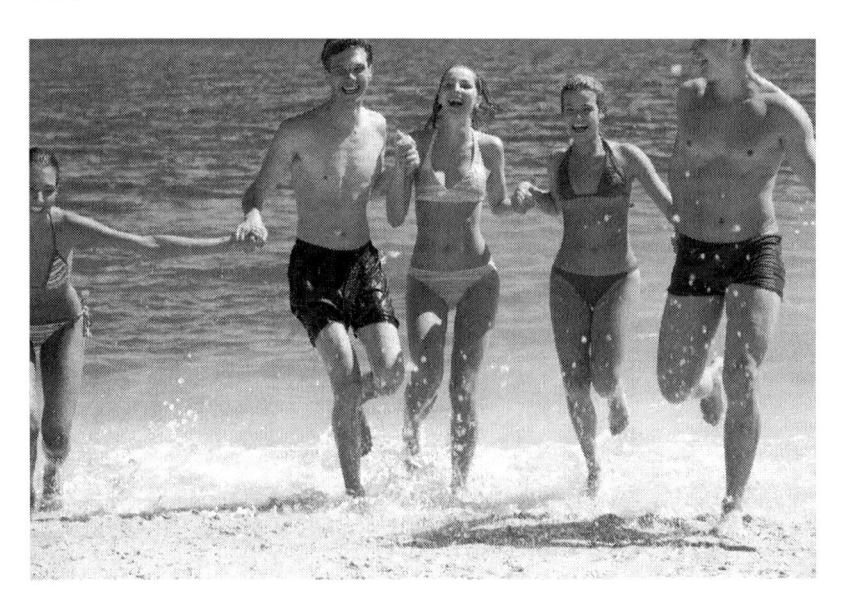

4. Visioning

4.1 Introduction

Most of the previous techniques are well known and mental imagery is used by therapists. With visioning, we are entering in an unexplored territory. However, visioning is the masterpiece of all the personal development courses.

4.2 Objectives:

Our objectives are :

- To show you how to define your vision and its "success image".
- To teach you the visioning techniques
- To give you some tips about managing your vision

By the end, you will know how to implement your vision in your subconscious. As a result, you will find yourself transported in a success story.

Real life example:

Universities and business schools ignore visioning. They do not teach how to implement success in your mind.

On the contrary, these techniques are intensively taught to sportsmen going to top competitions. Our educational public system trains better the sportsmen than the biz men!

4.3. Definition of Vision

The first and most important step for starting a business is to create your own vision.

Definition: Your Vision is what you want to become. Vision commits your personality. It answers the question: "what do you want to do with your life ? What is your mission ?"

4.4 How to discover your vision.

You have a vision. But you do not know it. You have to discover it in using a self analysis. Look at the following table. It shows that all our lives comprise activities that aim to satisfy requirements as in the table below:

Field	Activity	Requirements or aims
Physical	Exercise	Be healthy
Mental	Learn	Be educated
Social	Found a family Make friends	Love and be loved
Spiritual	Do good	Fulfill a spiritual mission

Using this model, try to complete the table. For example, it can be presumed that you are going to put in the mental field: learn management and be educated in business.

You will find yourself faced with a table that is yet too general. You have to go to the specifics. To do this, answer the following question: If I had unlimited money and time, what would I really like to become? (requirements or aims column). You will show in your table below your preference and just that.

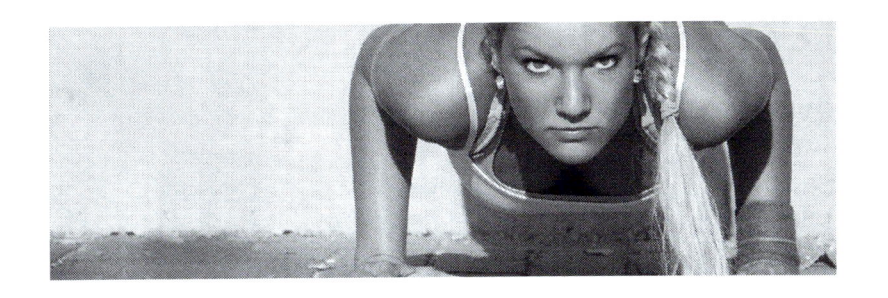

Field	Aim	Project
Physical	Live in the open air	
Mental	Knowledge of management	Manage a leisure business
Social	Have fun with friends	
Spiritual	Make my friends happy	

To help you, we will imagine the John's answers

This table, after a long self analysis shows the real aims of John. From these aims it is easy to deduce a vision. John is now able to describe his vision in one single sentence: I want to run a leisure biz to work in open air, have fun and make my friends happy.

That is a true vision. You will notice that we have not spoken about accumulating money. Money is not an activity in itself. It is a resource. We have not spoken about the investment needed to start a business. You need, for example, four off-road vehicles, a motor launch, diving equipment, etc. They are also resources. Resources here are not important.

Now, you have to do the exercise for yourself. You must obtain one single sentence for defining your vision!

4.5 How to Create your success image

Using your vision, you should now create your success image. The goal of the success image is to provide with a tool that you will constantly use for implementing your vision in your subconscious.

-Definition: The success image is once again a mental image, like the image resource. Instead of describing a past event that you had experienced, the success image describes a future event that you would like to experience.

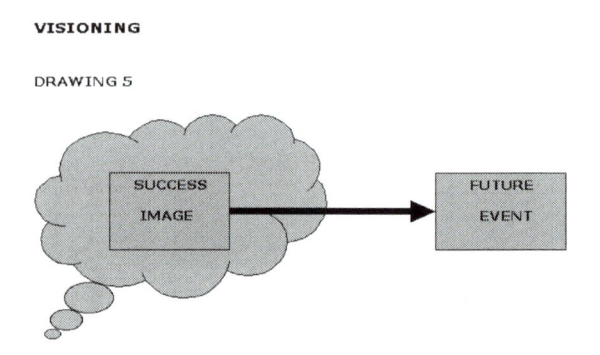

VISIONING

DRAWING 5

```
  ┌─────────┐          ┌─────────┐
  │ SUCCESS │   ──►    │ FUTURE  │
  │  IMAGE  │          │  EVENT  │
  └─────────┘          └─────────┘
```

The drawing illustrates this definition.

Important warning:

Don't confuse image resource, success image and remote viewing.

An image resource describes a past event that you had really experienced. For example, I had really experienced a pleasant promenade on the Thames river some decades ago!

A success image is a product of your imagination. It describes an event that you would be happy to experience in the future. For example, suppose that you are a little clerk. Your success image shows you acting as CEO of a big corporate. Of course, that is neither your past situation nor unfortunately your present. It's a fictitious image linked to your vision and your future.

Remote viewing is the ability to describe present event which are impossible to perceive with our sensory system. For example, remote viewing had been used by the CIA: People were trained to get a mental image of some secret bases in Siberia. It was the "Star gate program". It is supposed to have been cancelled by 1995 because of its poor results.

According to our John 's example of a vision, here is an example of a possible success image for John:

I am contemplating a magnificent landscape. I have led a team of customers and friends to the top of Mount Whitney. Glaciers are glittering. The snow is wonderful. I am exhausted but happy. I hear my team applaud me. I surf on an ocean of happiness and success.

As you see, the film should be neither too long nor too complex since you will have to repeatedly watch it.

You should now create your own success image: identify it and draw it. Once you have built your image, keep it in the smallest detail and don't change it any more. Our targeted ads could help you because they provide with images of happiness.

4.6 Visioning Techniques

You have now to implement in your subconscious this success image. That is the core job and once again it needs a bit of training.

1 The main process

For implementing your success image in the subconscious, you have to follow a precise process. First you have to relax as we have shown above. When you have gotten a full relaxation, you have to follow three sequences

FIRST SEQUENCE

The eyes are still closed. See your interior mental space as a black screen. Concentrate on this black screen taking at least five regular and slow breaths. Specify the outline of this area so that it resembles a blank television screen.

SECOND SEQUENCE

Imagine your screen turned on. To make this passage easier, make a habit of pressing together you thumb and index finger (anchoring), as though you were pressing your TV's remote control. This reflex association should make changing from one screen to the other easier.

THIRD SEQUENCE

Imagine the mental image of your success. For example, imagine the board of directors. You see your staff entering and leaving. Then imagine yourself coming in and sitting down in your President's chair. Everyone is looking at you and is waiting for your message.

The following drawing visualizes all this process:

DRAWING 6

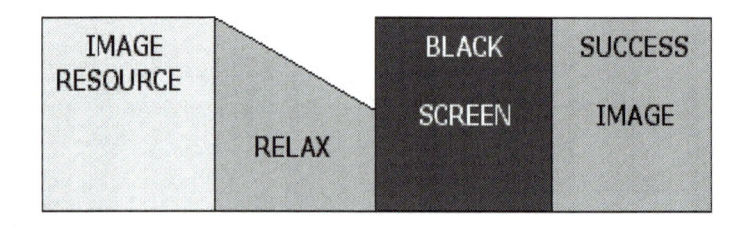

IMAGE RESOURCE	RELAX	BLACK SCREEN	SUCCESS IMAGE

It is important to properly visualize each detail: the boardroom's lighting, its shape, the colour of the furniture, the important people who are waiting for you and so on. This image must be mobile as on a television screen. Also imagine what you feel.

You will not manage such precision the first time or the second. The important thing is to keep the scenario chosen and carry out the exercise as often as possible.

In concrete terms, we recommend that you carry out this exercise every evening before going to bed. The more precision you gain at each exercise, the more this image will seem alive and the more it will happen in reality!

4.7 Supplementary techniques

The techniques described here will help you to deal with the difficulties of daily life. Just like with visioning, it is important to rigorously follow the procedure and practice as much as possible.

The specific vision:

You can use the same technique for special events: For example, you have a presentation to make tomorrow before a dozen people. Proceed in the same way as in the two previous stages.

For the third stage, imagine the meeting room and those present. You see yourself entering the room and starting to speak. The people listen to you with interest. Your presentation is a great success.

Using this training, you will manage easily to vision specific events and you will notice that, in most cases, events will happen just like you imagined them. This observation should encourage you to persevere in your general vision since it shows you the effectiveness of the method in your daily life.

The specific vision must always be coherent with the global vision. For example, if your vision includes a boardroom in a luxurious building, a specific vision of a sports race would have no coherence and would be completely ineffective. For global and specific visions to mutually strengthen each other, they must be part of the same world or scenario.

4.8 Take vitamins:

You take vitamins in the morning for your body, but you have to take vitamins also for your subconscious. For example, read the five quotes and create mental images associated with these five quotes and in coherence with your overall vision:

Closing your eyes, say them in watching the images associated with them each morning on getting up.

I feel sure of myself
Everything I do is easy
I am going to progress further today towards the aim that I have fixed myself
I had complete control over my future
Everyone helps me and likes me

There are your daily vitamins!

4.9. Managing The Visioning

1 Keep a log

Some of you certainly kept a diary when you were young. You should renew with this habit by keeping a log for your vision.

Obviously, don't include any negative experiences! Writing them down would just implement them in your subconscious in contradiction with your objective. On the other hand, describe in detail all your activities and thoughts from day to day concerning your vision.

Carefully note all the facts that seem strange, even if they are insignificant. For example, you meet a childhood friend you haven't seen for ten years by chance. Note this fact and think about it. It is surely a signal that is part of the realization of your vision.

Also note the sentences that you have heard during conversations that have attracted your attention without you knowing why. Your conscious doesn't know why but don't forget that your subconscious is working and that it knows. Analyze these sentences as though they were enigmas. You can find a hidden message for your vision.

Carefully note the dreams that you remember on waking up. Keep your log on your bedside table with a pen to be able to write them down straight away. Indeed, a few minutes after waking up, you will have completely forgotten them.

Regularly re-read your log at least once per week. You will be surprised to notice that strange fact get a meaning and that your action is developing quickly like a force that nothing will stop. Thanks to your training, your subconscious like an army of invisible hands is working for your own success, day after day!

2 Keep your way

You must absolutely maintain your genuine vision and its goals. Never downgrade it!

Along your course, the original reality is a magnet that holds you back. The vision is a magnet that pulls you forward and You are between them.

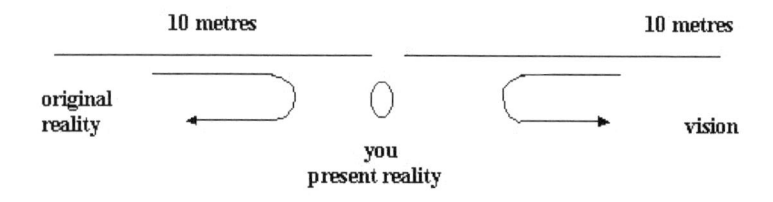

```
           10 metres                        10 metres
   _____          _____
original    ⎯⎯⎯⎯⎯⎯)   ○    (⎯⎯⎯⎯⎯⎯
reality   ←⎯⎯⎯⎯⎯                    ⎯⎯⎯⎯⎯→   vision
                           you
                       present reality
```

Let us suppose that, as in the diagram above, you are at an equal distance between the two. When you come across a difficulty, you will be tempted to lower your ambitions and downgrade your vision. Acting like this makes you think you are getting closer to the modified vision. You had 10 meters to run, you think that by limiting your ambitions there will only be 7 meters left.

This reasoning is false. Rather than getting closer to a vision that is easier to attain, you will on the contrary move away from it, as shown by the diagram below:

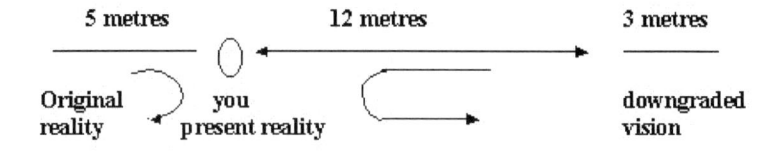

```
       5 metres            12 metres          3 metres
   _____   ○  ←⎯⎯⎯⎯⎯⎯⎯⎯⎯→   _____
                ⎯)                (⎯⎯⎯
 Original        you                          downgraded
 reality    ← present reality    ⎯⎯⎯→         vision
```

Continue with this way and your present reality will be again identified with the original one.

You must maintain your course at all costs. When a difficulty crops up, deal with it in a positive way.

To illustrate this fact that may seem obscure, we will take the example of a sailor. A weak breeze slowly pushes his boat towards his destination harbour: Athens. Suddenly, an adverse wind blows up. An unskilled sailor can choose to go towards the closest harbour.

In fact, an experienced sailor knows that he can use this wind as a lever. He adapts his sail. He beats windward and he knows he will reach Athens quicker than if he were pushed by a weak breeze.

4.10 Lesson summary

The first and most important step for starting a business is to create your own vision.

Your vision is what you want to become. Vision commits your personality. It answers the question: "what do you want to do with your life ? What is your mission ?"

Using your vision, you should create your success image. The success image is once again a mental image, like the image resource. Instead of describing a past event that you had experienced, the success image describes a future event that you would like to experience.

The goal of the success image is to provide with a tool that you will constantly use for implementing your vision in your subconscious. You have now to implement in your subconscious this success image. That is the core job and once again it needs a bit of training.

You must absolutely maintain your genuine vision and its goals. When a difficulty crops up, deal with it in a positive way. Never downgrade your vision!

Positive beliefs push reality towards the vision. The vision also pulls along reality. In the end, the reality must identify with the vision.

4.11 Do it yourself

1. You have to discover your vision and to write it in one single sentence.

2. Then you have to create your success image. Count about 15 hours for these two crucial tasks.

3. Once you have created your success image, you can begin the exercises for implementing it in your subconscious. During seven days, make the exercise 6 times a day. The next week, make it four times a day. Then, during the two following weeks, make it at least 2 times a day. It means that you have to perform 25 hours of intensive visioning within a month. Don't cheat! Remember that visioning is your key to success.

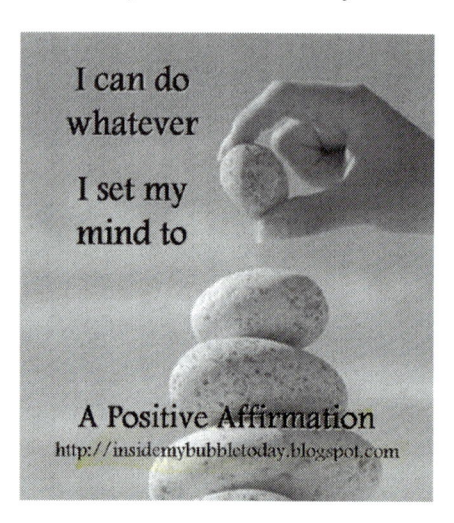

I can do whatever I set my mind to

A Positive Affirmation
http://insidemybubbletoday.blogspot.com

For the future, try to make one exercise every night before sleeping. When you are in trouble, make several exercises every days! Vision, vision, always vision!

4. Open a log and write down your observations.

Globally, these tasks represent 40 hours.

4.12 Business Creativity

1 Introduction

Right now, you have your vision and your success image implemented in your subconscious. You need an innovative idea and be sure that it will not be easy to find it! You must develop your creativity.

Business creativity is a core asset. No creativity, no new business! Fortunately, creativity can be improved through hard training.

2 Objectives

Our objectives are to teach you the main techniques for improving your creativity:

- We shall describe the different techniques.
- We shall underline those which are fitted for specific business goals.

Thanks for creativity and knowledge, you should get your business idea.

3. General Concepts

1. Definition:

Creativity is the process of bringing something new into being. This definition must be completed by a quote of the famous French scientist Poincare: Inventions consist in not making useless combinations but in making those which are useful and what are only a small minority. It means that it's not enough to produce new ideas. You must produce operational ideas and not dreams.

In our case, the true creativity is the power to invent and design products and services that will ensure the success of your company.

What is more, creativity consists in inventing what business you want and you are able to start!

Important warning

Do not confuse your vision, your success image and your business idea!

Your vision is a global aim of your life: It enables you to know if you really want to create a business and in what domain this biz could take place: For example tourism is a domain.

According to this vision, the success image is just a psychic tool for implementing your vision in your subconscious.

Then, according to your vision of working in tourism, you can have the idea to sell private islands. That is a real business idea!

What is more, business is constantly a creative activity and it's the only field where creative people can succeed. It is well known that very creative people are often persistent stubborn, and uncompromising! These traits are negative for a career as executive in a big corporate. On the contrary, a person who has absolutely none creativity could have very good chance to get high ranks in any big corporate or administration!

Real life example

Most administrations, many big corporates and a lot of high business schools should post yellow warning signals at every entrance, marked NO THINKING ZONE.

2. The creative process

Some people believe that creative individuals have inherited a lot of gifts and that they are talented or even genius. It's a wrong idea.

Creativity is not a matter of innate potential. As many things in life, creativity is the result of hard work and most of all serious training.

The creative process follows four different steps:

- Preparation: To train your mind.
- Incubation: To set back from the problem.
- Illumination: The idea arises in the mind like a sudden flash.
- Validation: You have to check the validity of the idea.

We can sum up this process with the following drawing :

DRAWING 9

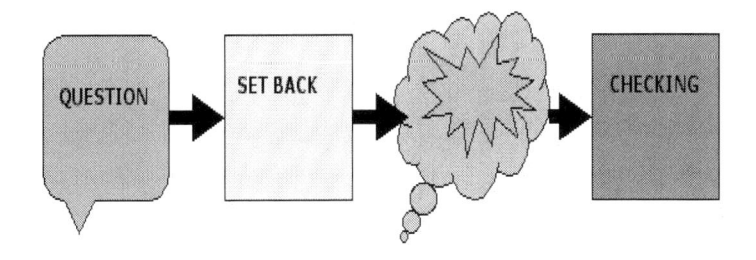

QUESTION → SET BACK → (illumination) → CHECKING

There are some other process but we shall adopt this one. The next reading will give you a history of the various views of the creative process, starting with the ancient greeks!

We shall now examine for each steps, what are the best appropriate techniques

2.1 Preparation

We shall distinguish long term preparation and short term.

1 Long term preparation

Just like for mental imagery and visioning we do not know the real cause of creativity but there are some basic preparations. We give you six advices:

Health: A creative thought depends on a well nourished brain. Since the beginning of history, some drugs are supposed to enhance the brain power. In the old times, it was mainly tobacco. Today, someone recommend to use serotonin and so on. Beware about these drugs. They can produce secondary effects and diseases (such as tobacco !).

Attention: Concentration and attention play a great role in long preparation: it means that you have to constantly think about your vision. You must think at it when you wake up. You must think at it in having lunch. You must think at it in playing tennis or golf. You must think at it before sleeping. To think constantly about the same thing is a good method for having innovative ideas about it.

Readings: In this course, we give you a method to improve your creativity but it must apply on a content. Readings of basic knowledge's provide with this content. Therefore, you will have to read carefully the lessons about economy.

Read everything and as much as you can. Reading constantly improves creativity because when you are reading a book, you always form a mental image of what is happening. As we shall see, mental imagery plays once again a great role in the creativity process.

On the contrary, Television does not train creativity and impoverish it because it shows the images and consequently there is nothing left to the imagination.

Real life example:

There is everywhere, even in developed countries, a lack of creativity. Of course, it's due to an ineffective education but it's also certainly due to television.

You cannot expect a great creativity of people who spend a big part of their time in looking at soccer games! Of course it's good for any political Power: Remember the Roman formula " bread and circus"!

To say the truth, the problem is not only due to the insipid content of television programs. It mainly results of the fact that television does not stimulate the imagination and therefore impoverish the creativity tank in the entire population.

External readings:

For your preparation, we suggest to make some creative readings in order to stimulate your mind. I don't ask you to become a worm book: You have just to visit "Global leader" on this site. You will find here several surveys which deal with new concepts.

Secondly, visit the "Spiritual odyssey". That is just pure creativity. We don't ask you to agree or not with the content but just to see how creativity is used. It's a very good exercise to stimulate your mind.

Meet people: Talk with friends and relatives and look at all sources of good ideas. You can get sometimes a word or an idea that could help you in starting the creative process.

Keep a log: Report immediately any idea you have in walking or in talking with everybody. Very often, a good observation of the streets during a walk will give you ideas.

Practice some exercises: To develop your creativity, we recommend the following techniques:

Relax. Close your eyes and imagine a familiar object: your dictionary for example. Turn the dictionary around. Examine it from above and from below. Change it's colour. Move it away as though it were 10 meters away from you. Bring it back closer. Give it immense dimensions then reduce it down to infinite proportions. Change its shape, turn it into a violin. Make it disappear and reappear.

This repetitive mental exercise should prepare you for the following exercises.

2 Short term preparation

Short term preparation means that you are going to have a creative session within a very short period. Consequently, you have to make some precise preparations. We give you three advices:

1. Choose a motivating environment:

The first thing is to choose an environment connected to your vision. For this purpose you have just to imagine it:

You have an office that is perhaps old and shabby. Imagine in the smallest detail the office in which you would like to work (lounge, leather chair, vast and functional desk etc.)

Each time you enter your real office, see your mental office. You will think more effectively.

Then Imagine your advisors: There are certainly people you admire: film stars, politicians etc. Choose two or three and put them in your mental office: They are now your advisors! Then imagine that you are talking to them. Imagine, their arguments.

Each time you have to carry out a creative session, go into your mental office and discuss the problems with your advisors!

2. Increase your intellectual capacities:

Top class swimmers imagine that their hands are twice as big as they actually are and that their feet are webbed. This vision helps swimmers go really faster.

Just before sleeping, make a relaxation phase and then imagine that your brain is bursting out of your skull and is forming a halo.

See yourself like this and you will gain in confidence in your intellectual capacities. Thanks to this new confidence, your capacities will really increase!

3. Control your breath:

we have seen in relaxation and visioning the role of the breath. Right now, we propose a more radical but very effective method.

One hour before the creative session, relax and hold the breath for as long as you can. Repeat this exercise and you will feel both a great excitation in your mind and a greater clarity.

4 Incubation

Incubation is a contingency phase: It means that you have not solved your problem during the creative session. Consequently instead to go on with the problem, it's better to set back from it. It's said that incubation can last minutes, weeks or years! we shall focus on incubation lasting hours and minutes!

1 Incubation lasting hours

An universal technique is simply to go to bed! Let 'suppose that you have a creative session and that you do not find any results. Stop and begin again to morrow. Very often the solution you were looking for is easily found after a good sleep.

2 Incubation lasting minutes

This incubation process takes place within the creative session. When you feel difficult to go further, just stop, go into a pause and make the following exercise:

- Call your image resource (A quiet river for example). Vision it and enjoy.
- Then, imagine again your mental office and your advisors
- You are now ready for beginning a second round of your creative session.

External readings

About preparation and incubation go to: www.enchantedmind.com . Visit the entire site. You will find some complementary explanations and a lot of interesting tests.

5. Illumination

We are now entering in the creative work and we expect to get an illumination. I like this word "illumination" because most often an innovative idea appears like a flash into your mind. It causes a great excitement and a feeling of happiness and pleasure.

We shall now review the different methods which are expected to provide you with this illumination.

1 Brainstorming

Brainstorming implies a group of person. In your case, as you are using creativity to get a new idea for starting your business, the group could include some friends and relatives.

The principle of any brainstorming session is that participants have to stimulate and inspire each other to create ideas. The purpose is to tap the subconscious mind of the members: One idea will suggest another idea trough the mechanism of association.

Participants should feel unrestricted but the ideas should be built on the ideas of others in order to facilitate the association and to use the subconscious rather than a conscious discourse. The more ideas, the better. None of the participants can criticize to any of the ideas that are proposed.

Creativity is expected to explode and to bring on the table a lot of exciting new ideas. In the final phase the ideas are selected, improved, combined and the group agree on a final working solution.

Real life example:

Brainstorming is the only mind method taught in schools and used on a large scale in continental Europe and overseas.

In the scholar environment influenced by Marxism, a "collective" process is always supposed to be more effective than an individual one!

Along my career, I have participated to many brainstorming sessions. I have never seen only one creative idea coming out from all these meetings!

In fact, the association of words does not work because the participants keep the control of their subconscious and fear to be ridiculous or simply to show their true nature. Consequently, the collective subconscious which should be the real motor of the exercise remains mute. People just bring a shopping list of conscious and reasonable ideas.

As we have explained in the history module (See global leader on this site and click on history module), creativity is a solitary work. New ideas are often difficult to communicate and other people generally react by discouraging it: "it would not work, it's a waste of time" and so on. When a group of people is involved, the final product is mostly a consensus that uses old and proven ideas. A consensus is quite the exact contrary of a creative idea.

Most discoveries are the work of one person. Of course large project require teams. In fact these projects are broken down into many small tasks and the best way to get creativity is to entrust only one person for each task.

Down to earth advice:

Thanks to Freud, Jung and so on, many psy underline the subconscious. We recognize this role and we have emphasized its power in the visioning process (See above) but it's not a reason to expand infinitely its virtues.

I think that a clear reason plays a major role in the creative process.

2 Mind mapping

Mind mapping has been invented by Tony Busan. In some way, it's like a brainstorming but with only one person: Yourself.

You take a paper and you write the subject of your research in the centre. Then, you start to think in at random in an inhibited style and you write all the ideas that come around the main subject. Then, for each specific idea you do the same and you write around all the ideas connected with. You rely all the ideas with arrows of different colours and you get the following result:

DRAWING 10

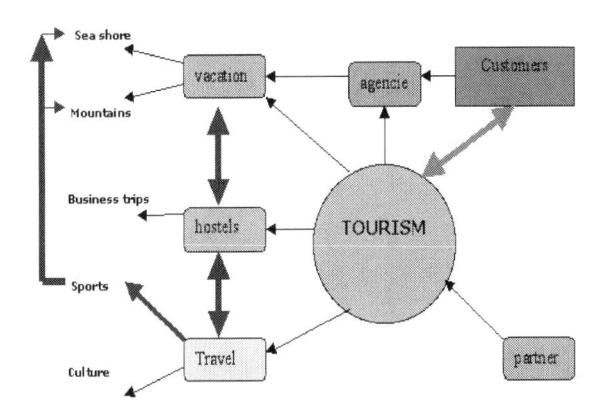

![Mind map diagram with TOURISM at center connected to: vacation (Sea shore, Mountains), agencie (Customers), hostels (Business trips), Travel (Sports, Culture), partner]

This map shows a research for discovering a business idea in the tourism field.

At first glance, the map only replaces the linear note with a more colourful and pleasant scheme. In fact, the principle is more subtle: The map is expected to reflect the real mechanism of the brain. It means that when you add an idea, you expand in the brain the connections between the cells and open new spaces of creativity. As you can see, the map looks like a network of neurons with their dendrites!

Real life example:

I use mind mapping for preparing a dissertation or for solving a problem. I don't use too much it for finding a new idea.

Mind mapping relies, like brainstorming, on the mechanism of association of ideas. On the contrary, I think that the real creativity must break off these associations which exist in our mind.

Nevertheless, we recommend you to use this tool.

External readings

Go to : www.mind-map.com . You will learn in this site how to use mind mapping. Read it carefully.

3. Mind revolution

For creative purpose, I use mainly that I call "mind revolution". You will understand the meaning of the word "revolution". It relies on three movements of the conscious thought:

Going to the extremes:

Facing a challenge, you have always to deal with six questions: Who, Why, What, Where, When and how. Dealing with these questions, try to see what would happen if things where going to the extremes. For example, what would happen if life time was infinite and on the contrary, what would happen if life time was only one day?

For example, Einstein developed the relativity by thinking what happened when matter travelled near the speed light. The laws of quantum theory rely on what would happen at the limits of small size particles. About business, you can ask what would happen if there is zero staff, or zero capital and so on.

Establish relations between things that don't have any:

Look for really absurd connections that no one would have thought of: Don't connect the image of your dictionary with a library. This is a normal relationship that shows no creativity. On the contrary connect this image with the hair of a person. The inventions of Archimedes, Leonardo de Vinci or Einstein were often based on connections that no one else would have thought of.

Deconstruct the thought: Most of our ideas or concepts are inserted in a group of ideas which are their companions and which prevent any creative thinking. Consequently, you must dislocate these current associations in order to find new ideas or concepts.

In the following drawing, I have two very usual connections. The blue squares show ideas connected to tourism and vacations. As long as I don't deconstruct the way of thinking, any idea of sun will bring an idea of sea or of sand and in fact I don't get any new idea.

Let suppose that I put a second series of ideas without any links with the former. In this example, the second series of gray squares illustrates ideas about justice, offence, trial, jail, convict, death penalty!

Now comparing these two series, I relate sea and jail and suddenly I get an illumination: I will sell private islands to rich people! You can see that in this tourism example, I get an immediate result! The idea may be stupid or useless. Anyway it's a new idea and I have gotten it in five minutes. (in fact this idea exists already!)

DRAWING 11

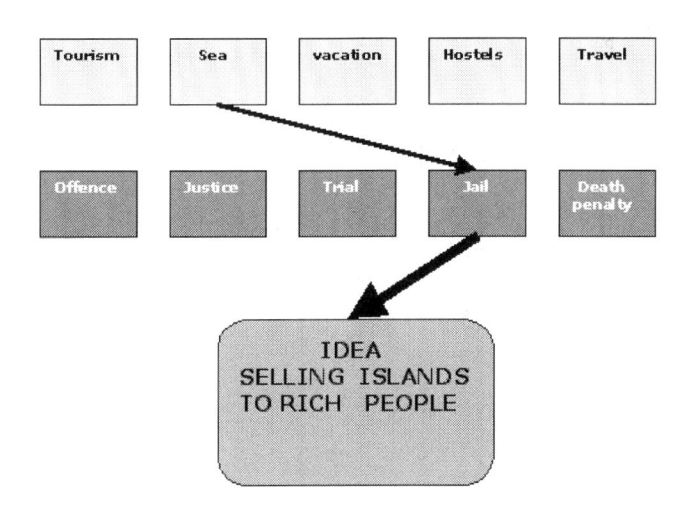

You can take notice that the process does not imply subconscious. On the contrary, it relies on a reasoning and on the will to dislocate current associations. In fact, I remove ideas from their normal statute and you understand why I call this process: "Mind revolution"! It's very easy to use with fast results.

External readings:

Go to www.mindtools.com . Click on "Creativity tools" and then on "Reversal", "SCAMPER", "Attribute listing", "Random input" and "Provocation". Each tool has its own advantages. You could observe some likeness between "Random input", "Provocation", and "Mind revolution". Nevertheless, each tool is different from the others.

4. Validation

All these exercises aim to produce new ideas. It does not mean that these ideas are worth or useful. So after the creative session, you must organize a validation session. In this case, it could be fruitful to call for a team because right now it's worth and useful to be criticized.

Down to earth advice:

Be very careful with the ideas you get very late in the night. When you find it, you are excited and they look very smart. Most of the time, too much coffee and tiredness explain these feelings.

On the next morning, when you read your notes, you often realize that you have just reinvented the wheel!

Discuss your idea with friends and potential customers: If you get interest and support, it means that your idea is innovative and that you can start the process of studying the project.

If your idea is a real technical invention, be very careful about its validation. Do not talk about it all around. In this case, be a discrete person and get a patent to protect your invention.

5. Lesson summary

Creativity is the power to invent and design products and services that will ensure the success of your company. In your case, creativity consists in inventing what business you want and you are able to start!

To think constantly about the same thing is a good method for having innovative ideas about it. In the creative process, focus on mind mapping and mind revolution.

In this course, we have given you a method to improve your creativity but it must apply on a content. Readings of basic knowledge's provides with this content. Therefore, you will have to read carefully the following lessons about Economy. Moreover, read as much as you can.

6. Do it Yourself:

We do not expect that you are right now ready for finding your business idea. You have to train your creativity but you must also apply it on a content because ideas need both creativity and knowledge. Maybe, you can have a first idea. Then, the learning of basic knowledge's should enable you to improve this first idea.

When you feel that you are ready and in a good mood, organize a creative session. It will need a half day. Use the tools that you have just learnt and try to get a first idea. It can just be a broad idea.

Count about 20 hours for four creative sessions. In fact, it's quite difficult to fix a duration. A good idea can mature a lot of time. On the contrary, It can be a sudden spark but it's impossible to say when it will happen.

Source: http://www.freeworldacademy.com/index.htm

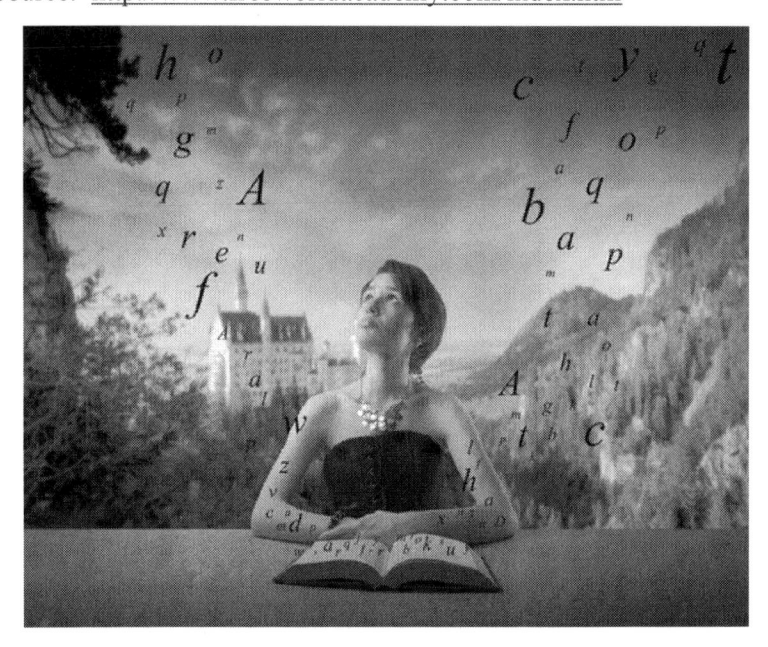

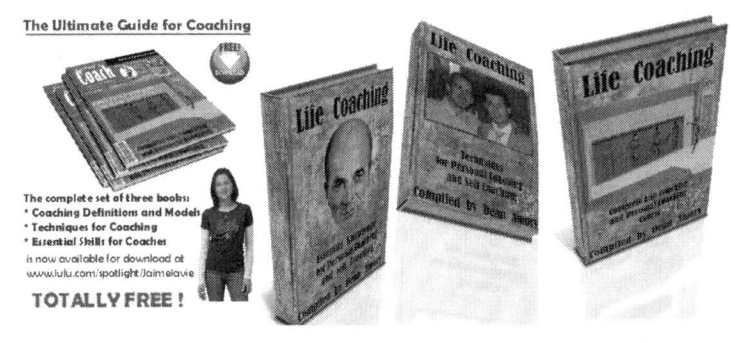

The Ultimate Guide for Coaching

The complete set of three books:
* Coaching Definitions and Models
* Techniques for Coaching
* Essential Skills for Coaches

is now available for download at
www.lulu.com/spotlight/Jaimelavie

TOTALLY FREE !

COMPLETE GUIDE FOR PERSONAL COACHING
Available for free download at http://www.lulu.com/spotlight/Jaimelavie

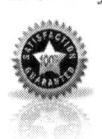

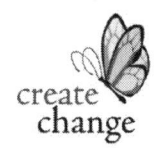

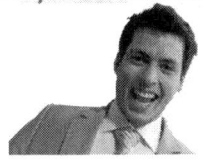

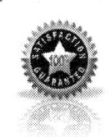

create change

5. Periscopic Learning aka Borrowed Genius

Win Wenger's Borrowed Genius technique is a creative thinking procedure that enables you to tap into the experience and knowledge of a self chosen expert in the field where you are looking for solutions or developments. To do so, move into the genius" body (mind) and experience things the way the genius would experience them.

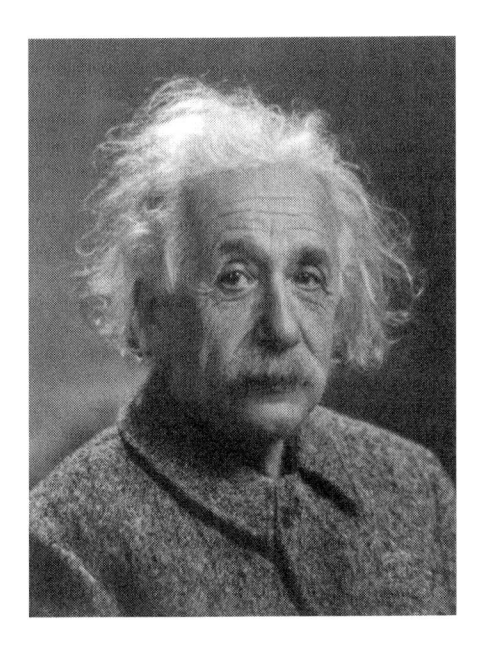

The key to this technique is that you describe what you see and experience OUT LOUD. The more you describe, the more details you will see.

If you are working with a partner, have him or her guide you through the different steps. If you are working alone, you might like to use a flow-chart or pre-record the steps for yourself, leaving plenty of time in which to explore.

Now choose the genius you would like to meet, the person who is a master in the skill or subject you would like to develop. The master may be someone you know or someone you don't know; may come from the past, present or future; or may be imaginary. You could also just let yourself be surprised by who or what your larger mind chooses to play the role of genius.

5.1 Steps:

Borrowed Genius Step One

Close your eyes and breathe deeply for a few minutes. Now imagine that you are standing in the middle of an exquisitely beautiful garden. Make this garden more beautiful than any you've ever seen. What colors and shapes do you see? What do you smell? Hear? Feel?

Borrowed Genius Step Two

Now invite your genius to join you in the garden. Whoever or whatever this genius is, begin describing them in the same rich detail you previously used to describe the garden. Make this genius completely real through the richness of your description, especially the feeling of their warm, welcoming presence.

Borrowed Genius Step Three

Imagine yourself moving forward and greeting your genius. Notice that your genius smiles at you and then turns so that their back is facing you. This is an invitation for you to step forward and move INTO the body of your genius.

Now start looking through their eyes, hearing with their ears, feeling with their feelings, and perceiving with their perceptions.

Observe the garden around you once again. How do "you" (as the genius) see it? Is anything different from how you saw it before? Whatever the differences are, make them utterly real as you describe them in all their richness.

Borrowed Genius Step Four

Now start doing whatever it is that your master is a genius AT. This may take you to another space where this skill is actually practiced, such as a concert hall where you are singing on stage or a laboratory where you are developing a scientific breakthrough. It might also take you back in time or into the future.

How do you feel when you're practicing your skill? What do you perceive? How does your body feel? What are your characteristic postures, gestures, patterns of movement?

Describe every sensory detail you can about HOW you (as your chosen genius) experience your abilities.

Borrowed Genius Step Five

Now begin to move freely through "your" memories. Go to the moment of greatest understanding or illumination, to your highest point or greatest aha! experience. This is the time when, more than any other, everything came together and suddenly made wonderful sense to you.

Describe out loud as much as you can of that moment and experience, particularly the perceptions and understandings you received.

Borrowed Genius Step Six

Now notice that you, the genius, are standing in front of a big, full-length mirror. Clap your hands once. The mirror has suddenly disappeared, and you and your genius have separated and are standing there facing each other.

Project a warm feeling of thanks to them and realize they, in turn, are thanking you for the opportunity to share with you some of the experiences that mean so much to them. Listen closely while your genius points out a key point in this experience or tells you something important about it that you've yet to realize.

Report your impressions regardless of whether they seem to make sense to you or not.

Borrowed Genius Step Seven

Finally, observe that your genius is handing you a cell phone, as you are handing one to them. With this exchange of gifts, you understand that you can access your genius' special knowledge, skills and abilities at any time, as he or she can access yours.

Now return with full awareness to the present, feeling refreshed, relaxed and confident. Spend some time writing down your experiences in your journal.

About Win Wenger

This exercise comes from Win Wenger, who is a bonafide genius himself and one of the leaders in the Creativity and Accelerated Learning movements. For more information about Win and his work—or to sign up for his free newsletter—go to: Project Renaissance AT http://www.winwenger.com/borrow1.htm

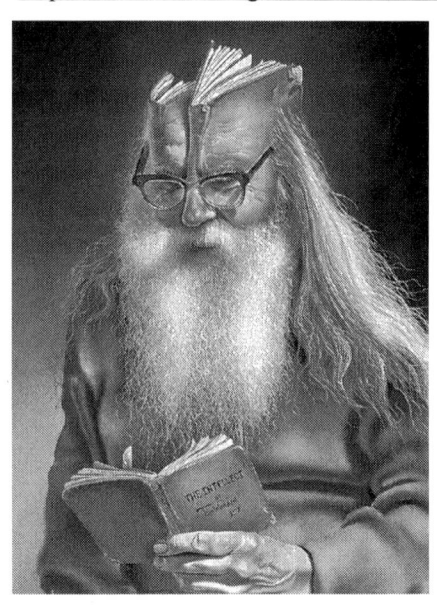

6. How to Be Your Own Hero

By Saleem Rana

6.1 "What do you want to be?"

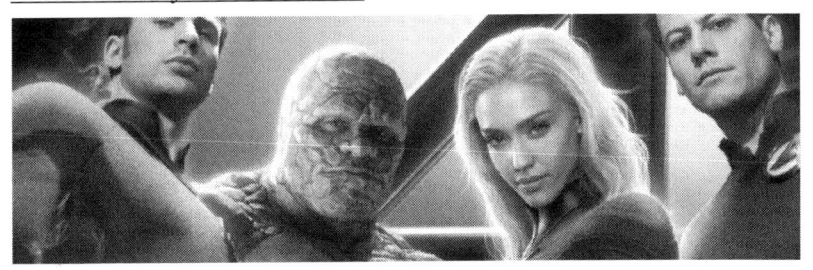

This is a deep question that we often ignore.

We are so busy caught up in making a living that we forget we have the power to design a life. We forget the possibility that at any moment we can turn everything around and become an outrageous success in life.

Most people opt for the default choice of mediocrity.

Yet this is not a pleasant choice. Nor does it provide more approval, control or safety than risking the idea of following your dreams. When you fail to aspire to be anything, your life rings hollow with the pain of feeling unfulfilled.

The main obstacle people encounter in following this line of thought is how to set it up.

While the dreaming and the intending can come to you with a little bit of effort to overcome your resistance, the challenge is in how to start.

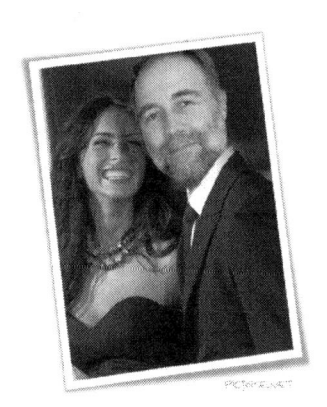

6.2 The Seven Success Steps

The truth is that you can be anything that you want to be—but you do have to work at it.

1) The first step is to have the courage to dream.

2) The second step is to make an intention (even if you don't have a clue on how to start).

3) The third step is to choose a role-model. Who is already doing what you want to do? Who is already the consummate actor, the best-selling writer, the charismatic businessman, the internet marketing millionaire, or the great humanitarian? Whatever you want to be—there is someone who is already an expert at it.

4) The fourth step is to study all you can about that particular person and that particular field of endeavour. You need knowledge…lots of it…you need to enter the arena mentally at first.

5) The fifth step is to emulate your role model. Adopt that person's habits and skills from your reading or even from your actual relationship with that person. Do what they do to have what they have—and when you do this, you'll be like or better than them.

6) The sixth step is to continue to study and practice. It's one thing to have the knowledge and to see how it is expressed in the form of someone doing what you want to do—and it is another to have it so deeply rooted into your subconscious mind that it seems like second nature.

7) And the seventh step is to persist. Obstacles will arise. Challenges will have to be faced. And you will have to work on your own disbelief that something extraordinary is possible for you; but if you persist long enough, you'll learn from your mistakes and become the person you really want to be, and do the things that you really want to do, and have the things that you really want to have.

Seize an hour today to dream your "impossible" dream. Over time, you will realize that nothing, in fact, is impossible.

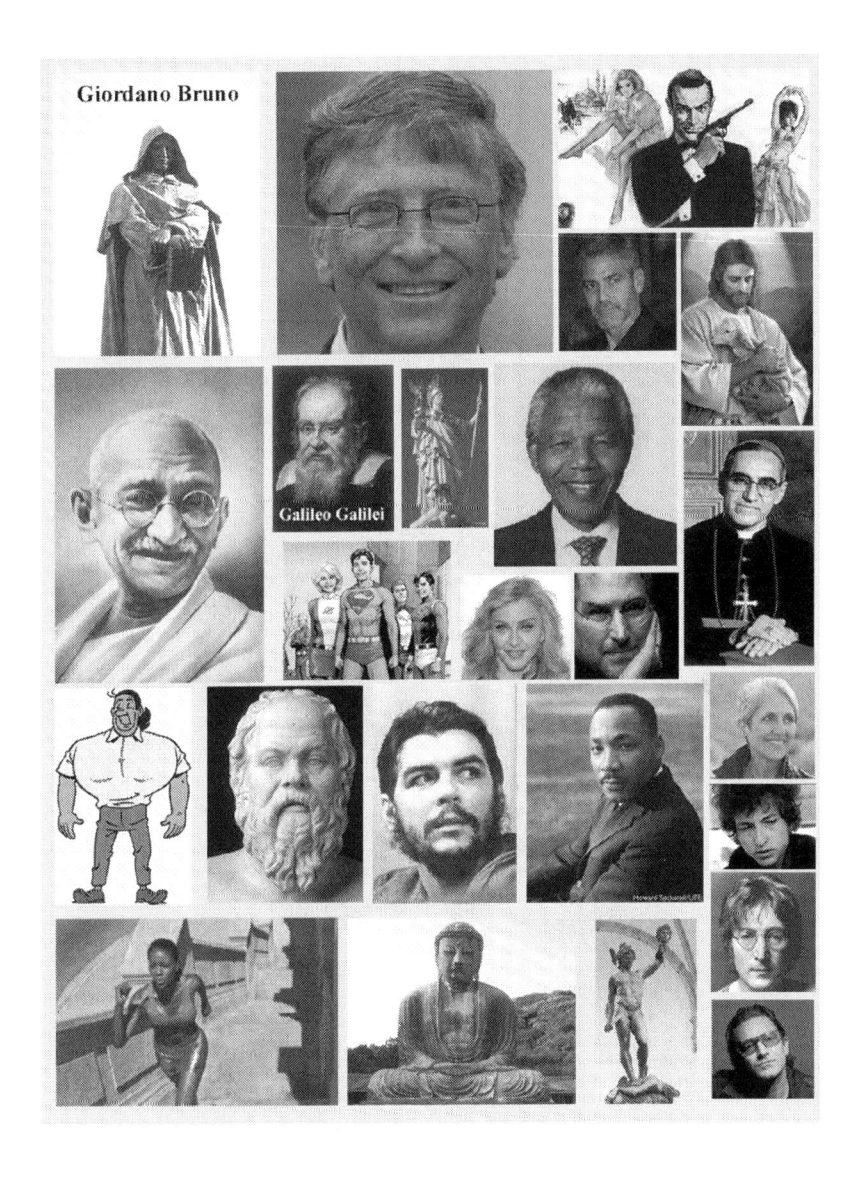

7. Positive Affirmations

7.1 The importance of positive affirmations

Negative thoughts often lead to feelings of anxiety, depression and an unhealthy state of mind. Practicing positive affirmations regularly tells your subconscious mind that you have the power to do what you need to do and make improvements to your life where it is needed.

Positive affirmations can have a direct affect on your energy level and overall well-being. When you focus on the positive, you give your mind and body a chance to feel energized, vibrant and focused. This state of mind makes it easier for you to build on your strengths and skills, let go of resentments or anger, and continue on your journey with less stress.

7.2 Some words are better than others.

It is important to find a combination of good words with a strong image. By putting the image-word message up at a place where you will regularly see it, the message that you are sending out to yourself will have an impact on you.

To reinforce the impact, it is good to read the words consciously several times per day and to commit to their meaning for you!

Remember what Aristotle said: "You are what you repeatedly do. Excellence is not an event -- it is a habit."

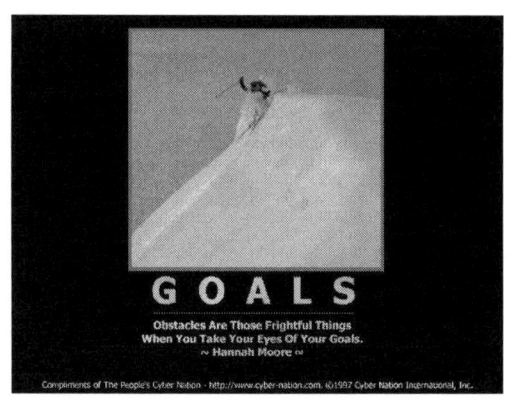

G O A L S

Obstacles Are Those Frightful Things
When You Take Your Eyes Of Your Goals.
~ Hannah Moore ~

Compliments of The People's Cyber Nation - http://www.cyber-nation.com. ©1997 Cyber Nation International, Inc.

7.3 What are good words for you?
There is Extra Power In Positive Words

- Power words that have special meaning to you.
- Words that reaffirm virtues.
- Healing words to overcome problems in your life.
- Words or phrases that motivate you.
- Special words to affirm your beliefs.
- Words that help you achieve who you can be.
- Statements or reminders of self belief.
- Words that promote positive thinking.
- Motivational words to promote positive growth.
- Mantras of building self esteem.
- Power thoughts to overcome negativity.
- Thoughts to inspire the best within you.
- Mantras to encourage self improvement.

Some words are stronger and more evocative than others. When you are on the phone with a prospect, you have about 10 seconds to grab and hold your prospect's attention. If you do not do that within that first 10 seconds, your call is more than likely over. If you get through that first 10 seconds, that buys you another 10 seconds. If you get through that 10 seconds it buys you yet another...and so on...10 seconds is not a lot of time. To get through those 10-second increments, you want to use the most powerful words that you have at your disposal.

If you are a beginner it is entirely possible, indeed even likely, that you may not be comfortable with certain powerful words or phrases. They may be very unlike your usual way of speaking. Even if you've been in sales for a while you might be set in your ways, accustomed to a certain delivery, and changing that might feel uncomfortable.

I've met many people who say they do not want to work with scripts because then they "cannot be themselves." Remembering that your prospecting call happens in 10-second increments, you want to be the very best self that you can be, every time. That requires preparation.

There are certain words and phrases that have a very powerful influence on the mind of the receiver. Professionals use key words and phrases in disciplines such as sales and psychology. They are employed to tap into the minds of those they want sell to, or to have influence over. They have an immediate and hypnotic impact on the mind, instantly gaining the attention of the listener. Used correctly they can ensure that the other person's attention remains locked onto you and the message you are trying to convey.

- Affirmations are strong statements of truth that has been achieved or needs to be achieved that a woman uses to control her destiny.
- Affirmations are positive and powerful inner thoughts and desires manifested in statements repeated to ones self.
- Affirmations are statements, the number of words isn't as important as the power of the words is what really matters.
- Affirmations are positive statements or powerful keywords that you think or say to achieve a result or strengthen a belief.
- The right affirmation can have a profound impact to make personal transformation in your life.

For positive affirmations to work and be effective each woman must feel they are empowered to impact her life in a positive way. These affirmation statements are powerful phrases like "I can change..." or "I will change..." they are not weak statements like "I hope I can change..." Or "I think I might be strong..."

Affirmations are based on "thoughts precede actions." Taking a quote from the Bible, "As a man thinketh, so is he." Proverbs 23:7. If something happens to make you happy it registers in your mind which can spread over your body in a positive way. However it all starts in your mind.

7.4 Free List of Positive Daily Affirmations

Abundance Affirmations
- I will live life abundantly.
- I will live the abundant life.
- The more abundantly I live the more abundance I will receive.
- I am prosperous.
- My live is prosperous.
- I am abundant.
- I am living abundantly.
- I am successful
- I know that whatever I put out comes back to me plentifully.
- I am a success.
- I am will be productive today.
- I respect my abilities
- I work to my full potential.
- I spend money wisely.
- I allow abundance to flow through me.
- I accept abundance today, tomorrow, and for my future.
- I accept abundance, wealth and prosperity in all its forms.

Dream Affirmations
- I am free to achieve whatever my mind can conceive.
- I have the power to achieve my dreams.
- I can achieve my dreams and help others achieve their dreams.
- When I help others achieve their dreams I will also fulfil my own dreams.
- I am not afraid to achieve my dreams.
- Dare to dream in life.
- Make your future out of your dreams.
- A life without dreams is not worth living.
- A dream is a positive way to look at your future.
- Dream all you want just don't get lost in your dreams but rather make your dreams a reality.

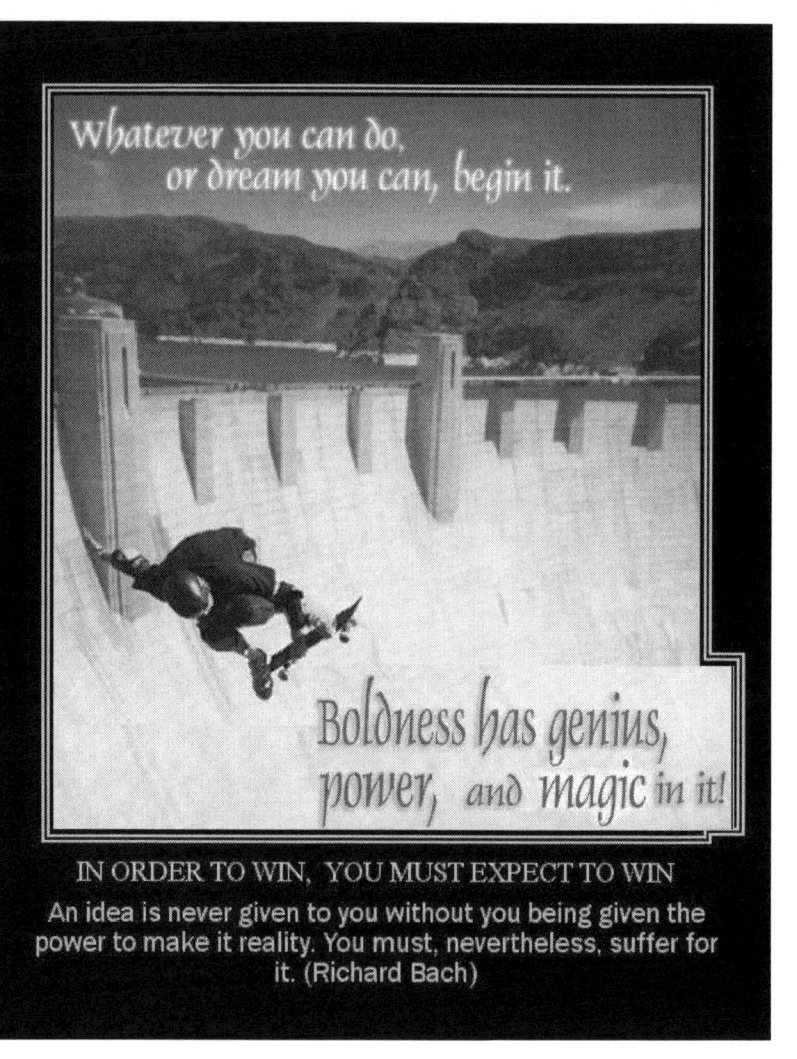

> Whatever you can do,
> or dream you can, begin it.
>
> Boldness has genius,
> power, and magic in it!

IN ORDER TO WIN, YOU MUST EXPECT TO WIN

An idea is never given to you without you being given the power to make it reality. You must, nevertheless, suffer for it. (Richard Bach)

- Dream it. Achieve it.

Success Affirmations:
- I enjoy success.
- I will have success today.
- I will succeed today.

- My possibilities are endless.
- My life is endless.
- My potential is endless.
- My accomplishments will last forever.
- A man may fulfil the object of his existence by asking a question he cannot answer, and attempting a task he cannot achieve. (Oliver Wendell Holmes)
- I avoid burnout by taking on only what I can handle today.
- I will prioritize my activities today.
- I will challenge myself today.
- I will change something about me today.
- I will manage my time better today.
- I will learn the lessons each day teaches me.
- I will handle my finances wisely today.
- I will take a risk to grow today.
- I will work hard and smart
- I am a winner.
- He has half the deed done who has made a beginning. (Oliver Wendell Holmes)
- I accept risk as a down payment on success.
- Today I will take a risk.
- Today I will seize every opportunity that comes my way.
- I will create positive opportunities.
- Taking risks is the path to growth.
- Problems are only problems when I take my eyes of my goals.
- Problems are simply stepping stones on the path to achieve my goals.
- I am a problem solver.
- I have the ability to handle problems.
- I can be a winner.
- I am a capable person.
- Never continue in a job you don't enjoy. If you're happy in what you're doing, you'll like yourself, you'll have inner peace. And if you have that, along with physical health, you

will have had more success than you could possibly have imagined. (Johnny Carson)
- I will enjoy the fruits of my labour.
- I worthy to be rewarded for what I do.
- I enjoy thinking.
- I succeed therefore I am successful.
- I will always be successful as long as I do what is right, true and moral.
- I will always be success if I believe in myself.
- I am a success because I never stop trying.
- Success isn't everything, it's the only thing.
- I have the energy to successful.
- My life is positive and successful.
- I define my success as (fill in the blanks).
- I am capable of endless success.
- If I live my life to my righteous standards I am successful.
- To reach a port we must sail, sometimes with the wind, and sometimes against it. But we must not drift or lie at anchor. (Oliver Wendell Holmes)
- Every positive effort I put out there, I will be equally rewarded.
- With positive thoughts and feelings in my mind I have created success.
- I am successful!
- I enjoy success everyday.
- I attribute my success to this - I never gave or took any excuse. (Florence Nightingale)
- The Keys To Success: Define success. Plan for success. Set goals for success. Sit back and enjoy the journey. Success is found along the way. (Callahan)
- It makes no sense that our caring, loving Creator would create us for failure, sadness or fear. We are destined to be creatures of success, happiness and fearless. It is our divine birthright to be successful, happy, fearless and strong. (Callahan)
- I don't know the key to success, but the key to failure is trying to please everybody. (Bill Cosby)

- Some of the greatest inventions and discoveries were made possible by mans ability to harness power and disperse it in a way that made great things happen. If you can learn to harness the vast energy and power of your mind and all the thoughts therein you can disperse that great power and you to can conceive and achieve great things. You can change the course of your life if you so desire. There are yet many things to discover, many things yet to be done, many things to teach. As much as mankind has achieved there remains much more to do and you could be in the middle of it all. (Callahan)
- Success is the ability to get inside your mind and stay there until you have figured something out, came up with a solution or just had a respite from the grind. Don't be afraid of your mind. He who is afraid of his mind will not achieve success. (Callahan)
- Success is what you define it to be. Know what success you want or you'll just be spinning your wheels. (Callahan)
- Want to get involved by blogging about free positive daily affirmations? Want to share some of your favourite affirmations? Create good karma? Check out our Positive List of Affirmations Blog. Part of being successful is sharing.

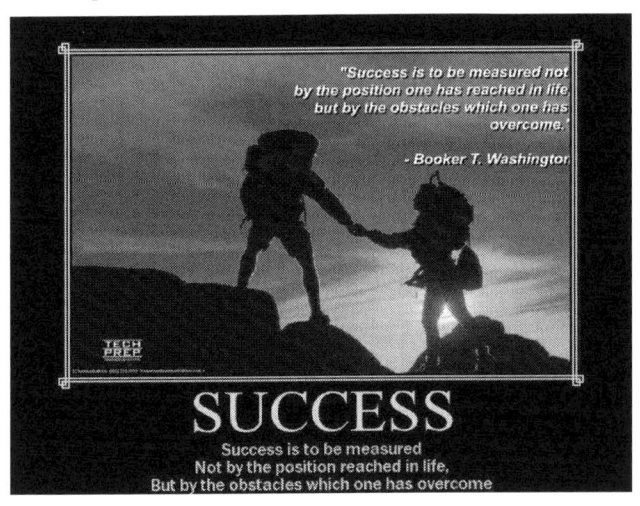

"Success is to be measured not by the position one has reached in life, but by the obstacles which one has overcome."
- Booker T. Washington

SUCCESS
Success is to be measured
Not by the position reached in life,
But by the obstacles which one has overcome

Prosperity Affirmations
- I can achieve prosperity in my life.
- I can have prosperity daily.

Love Affirmations
- I love therefore I am loveable.
- Love makes me happy. The I love the happier I am.
- I am a positive person filled with love.
- I love myself as I am
- Love is divine. I am divine. I am a creature of Love.
- Love comes from within me at all times.
- I love myself unconditionally.
- I accept love from others.
- The Universe has an endless supply of love. The more I give the more I receive.
- I am a loving person
- I accept the love of others
- I love myself
- I can show love by my actions
- I love my co-workers
- I love my neighbours
- I love my Wife
- I love my Husband
- I love my kids
- I am a lovable person
- I love living
- It's okay to love myself
- I love the opportunities in my life.
- The more I love the more I will be loved.
- I love everyone even though I don't always love what they do.
- Love is eternal. I love, therefore I am an eternal being.
- I pray that love will fill the hearts of those around me.
- Love makes me happy. The I love the happier I am.
- I love therefore I am loveable.
- I show love to all those I meet.

- I am worthy and loveable.
- I attract love into my life at every opportunity.
- Today I live with a strong sense of compassion and kindness to myself and others.

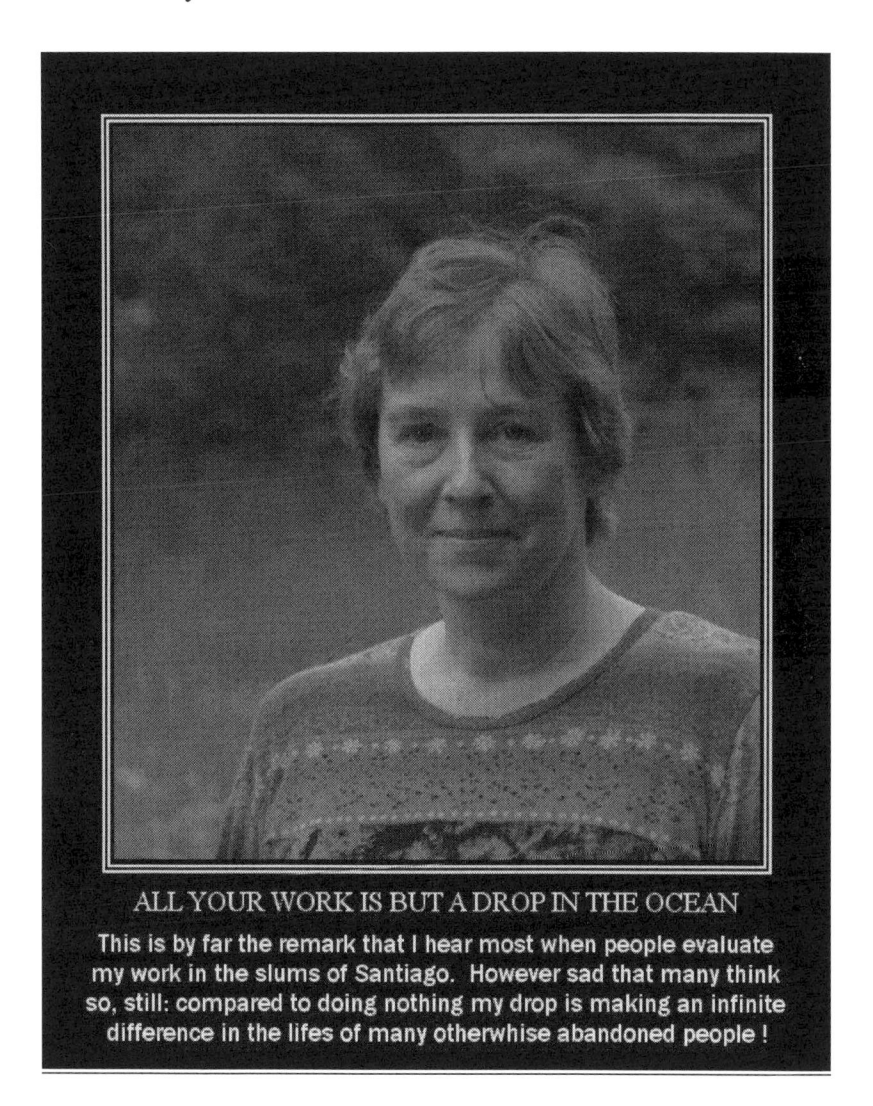

ALL YOUR WORK IS BUT A DROP IN THE OCEAN
This is by far the remark that I hear most when people evaluate my work in the slums of Santiago. However sad that many think so, still: compared to doing nothing my drop is making an infinite difference in the lifes of many otherwhise abandoned people !

Health Affirmations to promote a physical sense of well being.
- I am awesome.
- I have balance in my life.
- Every day my mind is filled with positive thoughts creating a beautiful life for me.
- I am beautiful.
- The Choice is within me.
- I have the choice to change.
- I always have choices!
- I am committed to excellence in everything I do.
- I am an excellent person.
- I seek excellence.
- I am loosing weight as I exercise
- I am healthy.
- I have vitality.
- I am loosing weight as I eat right.

Commitment Affirmations
- (I am committed to... (fill in the blank).)
- I am committed to a healthy life.
- I am committed to eating healthy.
- My commitment to exercise is real
- I am committed to loosing weight.
- I am committed to walking every day.
- I am committed to stop smoking.
- Commitment is my virtue.
- My commitment to … is eternal.
- I am committed to positive self talk.
- I am committed to be successful.
- I am committed to success in my life.
- I am committed to succeeding in my goals.
- I am committed to achieving my dreams.
- My commitment is to happiness.
- Commitment to my goals will bring success.
- Commitment is a powerful virtue.
- I am committed to happiness in my life.

- I am committed to sharing love

Happiness Affirmations

- Happiness is important to my physical and mental health
- I can have happiness in my life.
- Happiness is finding joy in the small things of life.
- I find joy in happiness.
- I can achieve true happiness by helping other to achieve happiness.
- Laughter is the best medicine.
- We do not quit playing because we grow old, we grow old because we quit playing. (Oliver Wendell Holmes)
- I am happy today.
- I am happy right now.
- I choose to resonate with happiness now, and for the rest of the day.
- Then there is a still higher type of courage - the courage to brave pain, to live with it, to never let others know of it and to still find joy in life; to wake up in the morning with an enthusiasm for the day ahead. (Howard Cosell)

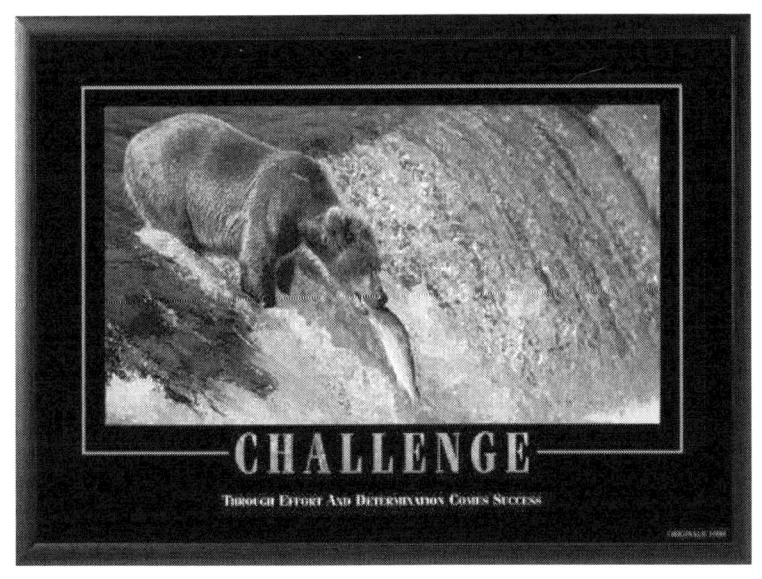

CHALLENGE

THROUGH EFFORT AND DETERMINATION COMES SUCCESS

Empowering Affirmations

- I am strong
- I am relaxed
- I have energy.
- I have inner strength.
- I am energetic.
- I am healthy.
- I nourish my mind, body and soul with positive affirmations.
- I heal quickly.
- I have powerful affirmations to control my health.
- I have control of my health and wellness.
- I have abundant energy and vitality.
- I fill the energy I need to do all the daily activities in my life.
- I am at peace.
- I have the courage to change.
- I control my body.
- I take care of my body and it cares of me.
- I can stop smoking.
- I can heal
- I will heal
- I will stop smoking.
- Today I will smoke less.
- Today I will control my temper.
- I will sleep easily tonight.
- I nurture my inner child.
- I love my inner child.
- I am in tune with my inner child.
- I embrace my inner child.
- My inner child is free to express myself.
- I will enjoy good health today.
- I will never take good health for granted.
- I am my own best friend.
- My family will benefit from my healthy changes.
- I will benefit from my healthy changes.
- I enjoy the beautiful things in my life.

- I am strong, focused and resilient.
- I give myself permission to enjoy success today.
- I give myself permission to be strong.
- I am in charge of my life and my mind.
- Today, I choose to be positive.

Relaxing Affirmations

- I feel calm and relaxed.
- I feel very peaceful and comfortable.
- I am enjoying feelings of contentment.
- I will benefit by relaxing more often
- I am in a peaceful but strong state of mind.
- I have inner strength.
- I am strong..
- My soul is strong.
- Because I am a woman / man I am strong.

Confidence Affirmations

- I recognize and appreciate my talents and skills.
- I am happy being the person I have become today.
- I accept and love myself, just as I accept and love others.

Affirmations for weight loss

- I accept my body as it is.
- I am losing weight for the healthy benefits.
- I make positive healthy choices.
- I love to exercise.
- I can't live without exercising.
- I exercise with passion.
- I eat wisely.
- I am thankful for healthy food.
- I love healthy food.
- I choose healthy food.
- I am fully satisfied. (Repeated after eating a healthy meal)
- I am full. (Repeated after eating a healthy meal)
- Weight loss is the result of using positive affirmations.

- Weight loss is the result of good choices.
- I make good choices.
- I take responsibility for my weight.
- I am in control of my body.
- I can loose weight.
- I am positive today.

Healing Affirmations

- I am making it through the day.
- Today is all that matters. (one day at a time concept)
- I will grow today in spite of the pain.
- I will smile today in spite of the pain
- I am blessed to have these experiences.
- I am happy today.
- I will shower today.
- I will get dressed today.
- This broken leg will only keep me down for a few months then I will run and jump and jump and run...
- Although my (Chronic Fatigue) "use whatever the illness in parenthesis" slows my body, my mind is free as a bird.
- My illness doesn't define me, my attitude and thoughts define me and they are good thoughts.

Health Quotes

- Every human being is the author of his own health or disease. (Buddha)
- The secret of health for both mind and body is not to mourn for the past, nor to worry about the future, but to live the present moment wisely and earnestly. (Buddha)
- Health is the greatest gift, contentment the greatest wealth, faithfulness the best relationship. (Buddha)
- To enjoy good health, to bring true happiness to one's family, to bring peace to all, one must first discipline and control one's own mind. If a man can control his mind he can find the way to Enlightenment, and all wisdom and virtue will naturally come to him. (Buddha)

- To keep the body in good health is a duty... otherwise we shall not be able to keep our mind strong and clear. (Buddha)
- Without health life is not life; it is only a state of langour and suffering - an image of death. (Buddha)
- Leave all the afternoon for exercise and recreation, which are as necessary as reading. I will rather say more necessary because health is worth more than learning. (Thomas Jefferson)
- Liberty is to the collective body, what health is to every individual body. Without health no pleasure can be tasted by man; without liberty, no happiness can be enjoyed by society. (Thomas Jefferson)
- Our greatest happiness does not depend on the condition of life in which chance has placed us, but is always the result of a good conscience, good health, occupation, and freedom in all just pursuits. (Thomas Jefferson)
- Even death is not to be feared by one who has lived wisely. (Buddha)
- Every human being is the author of his own health or disease. (Buddha)
- The secret of health for both mind and body is not to mourn for the past, nor to worry about the future, but to live the present moment wisely and earnestly. (Buddha)
- To enjoy good health, to bring true happiness to one's family, to bring peace to all, one must first discipline and control one's own mind. If a man can control his mind he can find the way to Enlightenment, and all wisdom and virtue will naturally come to him. (Buddha)
- To keep the body in good health is a duty... otherwise we shall not be able to keep our mind strong and clear. (Buddha)
- Without health life is not life; it is only a state of langour and suffering - an image of death. (Buddha)
- "I would rather know the person who has the disease than know the disease the person has." (Hippocrates)

Acceptance Affirmations
- I accept change.
- I accept who I am with joy.
- I accept others for what they are.
- Acceptance breeds acceptance. I will be accepting.
- I can accept myself for who I am.

Precious Affirmations
- I am precious to me.
- I am precious because of my self worth.
- Being a woman / man makes me precious

Specific Affirmations for Women
- My soul is tall.
- I celebrate my beautiful soul.
- My outer frame is what it is but my soul is gorgeous.
- I love myself.
- I am capable.
- I am proud of my body for what it is
- I only care about what I think of myself.
- What others think of my is their choice, what I think of myself is my choice.
- I have character.
- My personality traits are endearing.
- The lines and wrinkles of my outer frame show my history and character.
- Being healthy is more important than being a toothpick.
- I have power to change.
- I have wisdom to know what to change.
- My years make me wise.
- I have power to love and be loved.
- I can change.
- I am beautiful
- I can love without being in love
- I can be helpful without being used.
- I will change.

- I am precious in the eyes of God.
- I have power to choose my course in life.
- I have unique attributes and abilities because I am a Woman.
-

ENJOY ALL YOU DO

WHAT MUST BE DONE, MUST BE DONE.
YOU MAY AS WELL DO THINGS WITH A SMILE.

Positive Affirmations
- My inner strength and joy come from within myself.
- I am flexible and ready for opportunities when they arise.
- My intuition, or spirit, guides me in making decisions that are beneficial for myself and for others.
- Heaven provides plenty of opportunity for love and abundance.
- The more I give, the more I receive.
- I am a caring person.
- I have faith in myself.
- I love the sinner, not the sin.
- I love the potential in people.
- I love the virtuous opportunities the world has to offer.

Believe Affirmations
- I believe in myself.

Best Friends Affirmations
- Best Friends make the world go round.
- I treat my Friends as a gift from God.
- Friendship Affirmations
- Friendship is the best gift to give and to receive.
- It's better by far at the rainbow's end to find not gold, but the heart of a friend.

Beautiful Affirmations
- I am beautiful.
- Life is beautiful.
- My beauty lies within.
- All beautify starts from within.
- Where there is love there is beauty..

Cheer Affirmations
- I am cheerful.
- I need to have Cheer in my life.
- I will be of good Cheer.

Courage Affirmations

- I have the courage needed to change myself for the better.
- I have courage to stand up for myself.
- I have courage.
- I have the courage to do what is right
- I have courage to choose the right choices.
- Courage is my foundation.
- I have the courage to succeed.
- I have courage to get out of bed this morning.
- I have courage to do what is right.
- I have the courage to accept that I need the help of my Creator.
- Courage is a virtue that does not make me mean or heavy handed.
- I have the courage needed to change myself for the better.
- I have courage to stand up for myself.
- I have courage.
- I have the courage to do what is right
- I have courage to choose the right choices.
- Courage is my inner foundation.
- I have the courage to change.
- I have the courage needed to forgive.
- I have the courage to live.
- I am brave.
- I can bravely meet life's challenges.
- Bravery is a virtue within me.

Destiny Affirmations

- My destiny is to be the best I can be.
- Wealth is my destiny
- Good health is my destiny
- Success is my destiny
- Greatness is my destiny
- My destiny comes from within.
- Freedom Affirmations

- I have the freedom to choose for myself.
- No one can take my personal freedom from me.
- My freedom comes from within.

Joy Affirmations

- I find joy when I am not critical of others
- I am a joyful person.
- I will have joy today.
- I will be joyful today.
- I will find joy in the silly things of life.
- Today I affirm my joy.
- I find joy in friendships.
- My joy comes from love.
- My joy comes from within myself.
- I am joyful
- I find joy in being open with my friends.
- I have the power to be joyful.
- Joy comes from my positive mental attitude.
- Today I will be filled with joy about my life.
- Today I am full of joy.
- Today I will be filled with joy about the things that surround me and accepting of the things I have not control over.
- If at the end of the day you have not found joy or happiness perhaps you were not paying close attention.
- I know that today's discouragement will be replaced by tomorrow's joy.
- I enjoy life

Passion Affirmations

- I have passion to reach my divine potential.
- I am a passionate person.
- I have passion for life.
- I have passion for peace, harmony and truth.

Patience Affirmations
- I can have patience while improving myself to reach my potential.
-

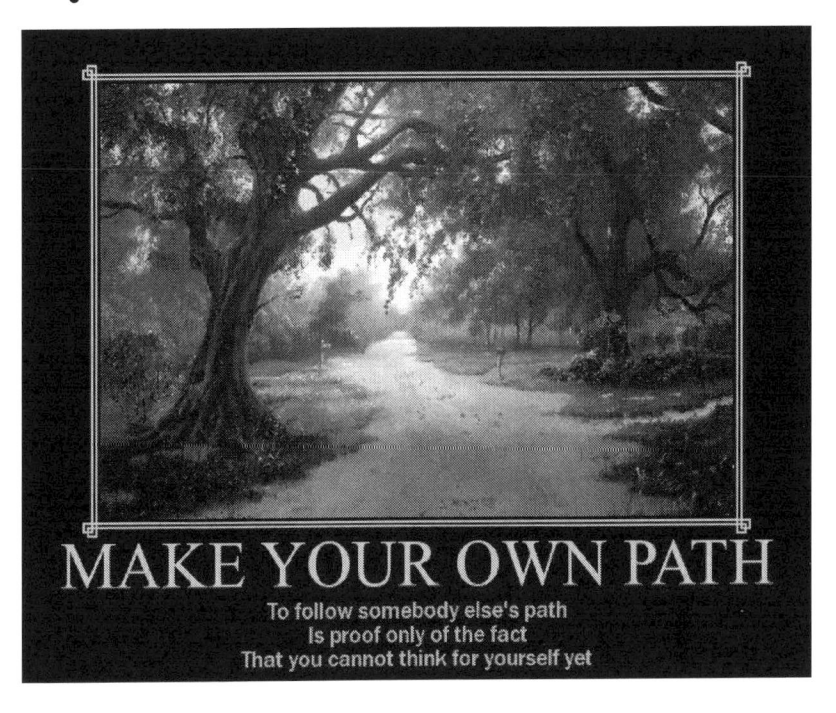

MAKE YOUR OWN PATH
To follow somebody else's path
Is proof only of the fact
That you cannot think for yourself yet

Peace Affirmations
- I am a peaceful person.
- I can have peace in my life.
- The peace in life you seek starts within yourself.
- To achieve outer peace first achieve inner peace.
- I can heal myself by thinking peaceful thoughts, I can help to heal others by saying peaceful words, and to do treat others peacefully.
- I can allow the spirit of peace to feel my soul.

- Peace is not just the absence of conflict, it is a soul filled with love, joy, happiness, patience, truth, harmony and serenity.
- I have passion for peace, harmony and truth.
- Where there is peace there is beauty.
- I am at peace with myself.
- I am at peace with the world
- I accept peace, joy and serenity in my life.
- I embrace a peaceful, relaxed and joyful state of mind.
- I can let go and enjoy peacefulness today

Perfect Affirmations

- I can become perfect one step at a time.

Responsibility Affirmations

- I have the divine responsibility to be the best I can be.

Serenity Affirmations

- I will let the spirit of serenity fill my soul.
- I can achieve serenity daily.

Teamwork Affirmations

- Teamwork makes the impossible possible.

Willingness Affirmations

- A willingness to live, to love, to serve, to care and forgive is the essence of the abundant life.
- I have a willingness to change.

Wisdom Affirmations

- Wisdom is learned by living life with your eyes open and not repeating the mistakes of the past.
- Wisdom is learning from others mistakes and not repeating them.
- I am wise.

Hope Affirmations
- Each day I hope for the best and achieve what I can.
- I can reaffirm Hope by being positive.
- Being hopeful helps to allow the spirit of hope to fill my soul.

Discipline Affirmations
- I have the discipline to make changes in my life.
- With discipline I will achieve my goals.
- With discipline I will achieve my dreams.

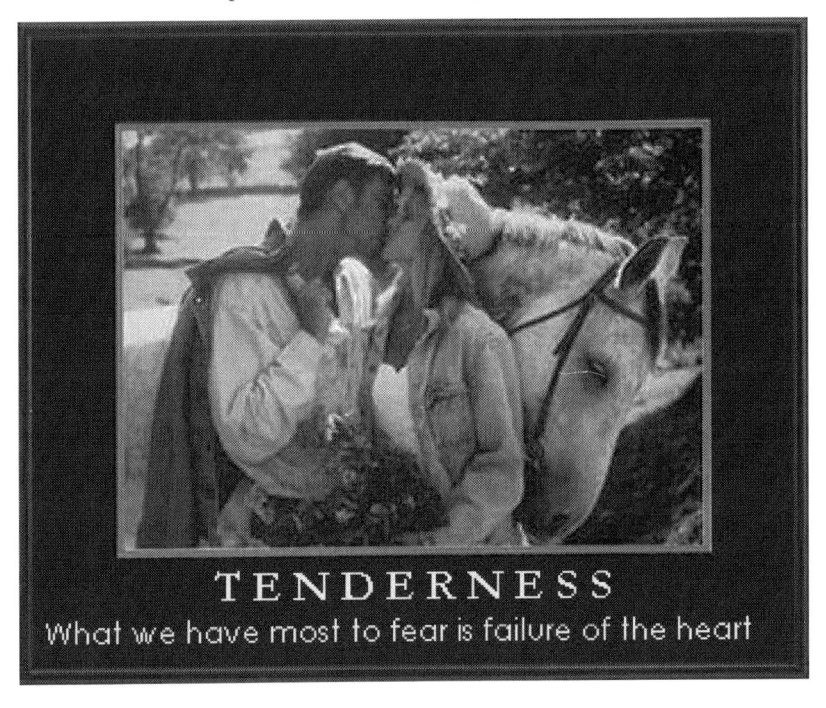

TENDERNESS
What we have most to fear is failure of the heart

Motivation Affirmations
- I am motivated to change.
- I am motivated to find peace.
- I have motivation to live with harmony and balance.
- I have the motivation to be the best I can be.

Power Affirmations
- I have the power within me to change.
- I have power to be the best I can be.
- I have the power to have harmony.
- I have the power to achieve serenity.
- No one is more powerful than the humble.

Fairness Affirmations
- I am committed to fairness in all my actions.
- I will be fair to everyone I come in contact with.

Harmony Affirmations
- Peace comes from harmony.
- I will live my life in harmony.
- I can allow the spirit of harmony to find rest in my soul.
- I cannot achieve harmony, serenity, peace or joy in my life without treating others in such a way to help them achieve the same.

Help Affirmations
- A helping hand is the best gift to give.
- I have the ability to help others.
- I can find joy in helping others.

Life Affirmations
- Life is what your thoughts will let it be.
- I will live life to its fullest.
- I love life.
- Life is only what I make out of it.
- I will live my life to exceed my potential.
- Positive affirmations help me to live life to my full potential.

Open-Minded Affirmations

- I am open-minded.
- I am open-minded to consider others opinions.
- I am open-minded to other cultures.
- I am open-mined to other ways of thinking.

Respect Affirmations

- I respect myself.
- I respect others.

Smile Affirmations

- A smile is the gift where the more you give the more you receive.
- Sharing a smile is a gift to all who look at you.
- Give the gift of a smile.
- Lift someone's burdens with a smile.

Sincerity Affirmations

- I can expect sincerity only when I am sincere.
- I will be sincere.

Trust Affirmations

- I choose to be trustworthy.
- I can be trusted.
- I am trustworthy.
- I will trust my intuition.
- My intuition is worth trusting.

Survivor Affirmations

- I am a survivor.
- The power to survive is within me.
- I have the strength to survive.

Wonderful Affirmations

- It's up me to make things wonderful.
- My life is wonderful.
- Life is wonderment.

Faith Affirmations

- I have faith in myself.
- I have faith in my better self.
- I have faith in the goodness of life.

Forgiveness Affirmations

- I can and will give forgiveness to to others.
- I have the power to forgive.
- I will forgive
- I will forgive myself.
- I will be at peace when I forgive others
- Today I will forgive.

Wish Affirmations

- A person without a wish is a person void of life.

Vision Affirmations

- Life without vision is no better than a fish in a fish bowl.
- I have a vision.
- I can achieve my vision.

Source:

09/15/2012   HandCraftedCollectibles.Com

Copyright 2002 - 2012

HandCraftedCollectibles.Com:

125 East Main Street, Suite # 212, American Fork, UT 84003

This page is Copyright protected. Permission is granted to use any quotes from this page only if a direct link to this page is used along with the quote(s). If the quote(s) is desired for print use then a reference to this page (URL) must be used for credit.

Bookmark or add to your favorites this web page which is your primary source for positive daily affirmations.

http://www.handcraftedcollectibles.com/positive_affirmations.htm

8. Animal Totems

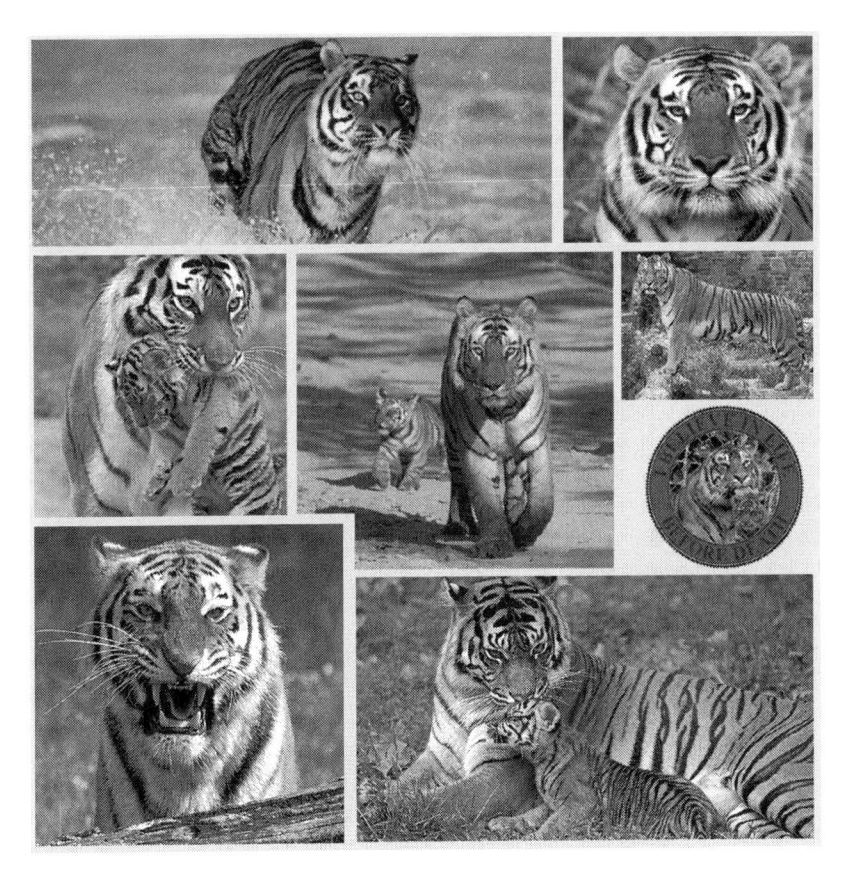

8.1 I am the Tigress

The tigress is strong, bold, unwavering and extremely quick and accurate. She's a very clean animal, whose hearing is her most highly developed sense and she is far more dependent upon hearing than sight or smell.

She is dedicated to the high ideals of loyalty, courage, endurance and heroism. She is willing to put herself in herms way to do what is right, confident in her ability to triumph. The tigress is a beast that prefers solitude. While she's very protective of her cubs and willing to share her kill with them and the father, she does not take too kindly to other tigers from intruding on her turf. She is neither dependant on the tiger nor subservient to him. She decides if she wants to let him share the kill or not.

So if you have a tigress in you, you're a team player even as you still retain your individuality. You don't brook any nonsense, from your co-workers or your superiors. You are a quick and accurate worker and demand acknowledgement for your achievements. You know that you can do anything as well as anybody else, even when you're smaller in size.

Source:

http://jobsearchjungle.com/blog/?tag=characteristics

Carolyn Thompson

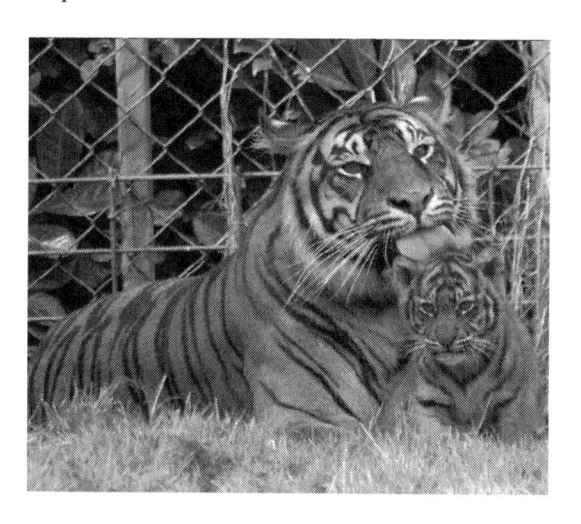

8.2 Discover Your Personal Totem

Animal totems contain a natural power that can allow you to see and love and know more of the earth, life and especially yourself.

Animal spirit guide totems hold power and knowledge that we can use to be one with nature - all that is and will be. Many cultures of the past understood and used the power of animal totems.

Totems can be particularly useful in today's society where it is easy to forget the essence and true spirit of life and love in the midst of high technology. Use your personal animal totem to awaken the natural balance with nature that you already possess. You can be healthier and happier physically, mentally, emotionally, and spiritually in understanding and honouring your animal totems.

How to find your personal totem

- There are several ways to know what your animal totem is.
- You may feel so attracted to a certain animal that you have collected many drawings, carvings or other types of images of this animal. The likeness of the animal brings the animal and its powers closer to you.
- There may be an animal that frightens you. This could be your animal totem if there are lessons you should learn that you are strongly resisting.
- You may dream about the same animal over and over.
- The animal may come to you in deep meditation.
- You may feel strongly about one of your zodiac animals, birth zodiac, Chinese zodiac.

However you find your animal totem you are sure to have a changed life if you listen and learn the lessons of your animal spirit guide!

8.3 Associations linked to some animals

When choosing an animal totem, be specific: there are huge differences in associated images between a pitbull, a german shepherd and a St Bernhard

Animal Totem Significance

(Most popular "Lifetime" Totems)

EAGLE – "Spirit" – ILLUMINATION: The Higher Mind and creative force of the Great Spirit.

HAWK – "Messenger" – INTUITION: Being aware of life's signals and receiving them.

ELK – "Stamina" – WARRIOR: Realigning the Self with group consciousness.

DEER – "Gentleness" – COMPASSION – Healing power of gentleness that touches all hearts.

BEAR – "Inner-Knowing" – INTROSPECTION – Strength of achievement that comes from intuition.

SNAKE – "Transmutation" – ALCHEMY - Transformation through thought, action or desire.

SKUNK – "Reputation" – DISTINCTION – Assertion without EGO and self-respect.

OTTER – "Woman Medicine" – FEMALE ENERGY – Healthy curiosity and living life without preconceptions and suspicion.

BUTTERFLY – "Transformation" – CYCLES – Going within to bring fruitfulness without.

TURTLE – "Mother Earth" – PROTECTION – Roundedness and observing all situations with compassion.

MOOSE – "Self Esteem" – PROGRESS - Joy without EGO in accomplishment.

PORCUPINE – "Innocence" – TRUST – Faith in the Divine Plan.

COYOTE – "Trickster" – MASTERY – Consciousness that is born from folly.

DOG – "Loyalty" – PHILANTHROPY – Loyalty and service that is not countermanded by need for approval.

WOLF – "Teacher" - WISDOM – Sharing of the Higher Truths.

RAVEN – "Magic" – WIZARDRY – Trusting the power of the unknown and the Great Mysteries.

MOUNTAIN LION – "Leadership" – CONFIDENCE – Balancing intention with physical strength and grace.

LYNX – "Secrets" – CLAIRVOYANCE – Paying attention to revelations and using caution about what you reveal.

BUFFALO – "Prayer and Abundance" – SUSTENANCE – The power of prayer and reconnecting to the meaning of life and the value of peace.

MOUSE – "Scrutiny" – METHODOLOGY – There is always more to learn.

OWL – "Observation" – TRUTH – Speaking the whole truth rather than half truths or lying by omission. The power of keen "silence" to intuit life situations.

BEAVER – "Builder" – TEAMWORK - Sense of community achieved through collaboration.

OPOSSUM – "Diversion" – STRATEGY – Mental and physical prowess that leads to progress.

CROW - "Law" – SUPERNATURAL - Sacred Law. Knowledge of alchemy. Shape shifting. Higher Order of Right and Wrong.

FOX – "Camouflage" – CUNNING – The sly power behind ingenious manoeuvres.

SQUIRREL – "Gathering" – PRESERVATION – The ability to prepare and honour the future.

DRAGONFLY – "Illusion" – ENLIGHTENMENT – Things are never completely as they seem.

ARMADILLO – "Boundaries" – SHEILD – Defining one's space.

BADGER - "Aggressiveness" – ACCOMPLISHMENT – The "BOSS"… the one who gets things done.

RABBIT – "Fear" – WORRY – Learning to resist pessimism and being attached to negative outcomes.

TURKEY – "Give-Away" – SELFLESSNESS – "Doing unto others." All life is Sacred.

ANT – "Patience" – COMMUNITY-MINDEDNESS - Working for the good of the whole.

WEASEL – "Stealth" – ACCURACY – The hidden reasons behind anything.

GROUSE – "Sacred Spiral" – VISION – The spiralling DNA double helix. The Divine treatment of motion.

HORSE – "Power" – FORTITUDE – True power is the wisdom found in remembering your total journey.

LIZARD – "Dreaming" – MANIFESTATION – Understanding the shadow side of reality where dreams are reviewed before being manifested physically.

ANTELOPE – "Action" – MOVEMENT - Honouring destiny by masking the decision to start moving.

FROG – "Cleansing" – PURIFYING – Purging the self of distractions, guilt, frustrations and emptiness.

SWAN – "Grace" – RHYTHM – Surrendering to the grace of the rhythm of the Universe and altered states of awareness.

DOLPHIN – "Manna" – LIFE FORCE – Linking to the Great Spirit. Answers to questions. Patterns of Divine energy.

WHALE – "Record Keeper" – AKASHA – Frequencies in DNA codes. Exploring the Soul's personal records.

BAT – "Rebirth" – GROWTH – Symbolic death that paves the way for the new "self."

SPIDER – "Weaving"- FATE – Connection to the primordial. Creation and expansiveness of the Eternal Plan.

HUMMINGBIRD – "Joy" – FREEDOM - Paroxysms of joy and renewal in the magic of living.

BLUE HERON – "Self-Reflection" – SELF WORTH – Discovering the role of spiritual essence and Divine purpose.

RACCOON – "Generous Protector" – DEFENDER – Vigilance. Standing up for the underdog. Honour.

PRAIRIE DOG – "Retreat" - BASICS – Pushing too hard can create resistance.

WILD BOAR – "Confrontation" – COURAGE – Honouring the truth, confronting fears, facing challenges.

SALMON – "Inner knowing" – RESOURCES – Reflection and reclaiming the inner self. Discernment and authentic vision.

ALLIGATOR – "Integration" – FLOW – Right of passage. Seeing all sides of a situation and not passing judgment but making decisions.

JAGUAR – "Impeccability" – HONOR – Maintaining integrity and holding on to forthrightness and honesty.

BLACK PANTHER – "Embracing the unknown" – SHADOW SELF – Trusting in the future and the mysteries of life. Letting it BE. Self discovery and healing processes.

Sources:

http://crystal-cure.com/totem-questionnaire.html

http://www.lightforcenetwork.com/group-content/lifetime-animal-totems

145

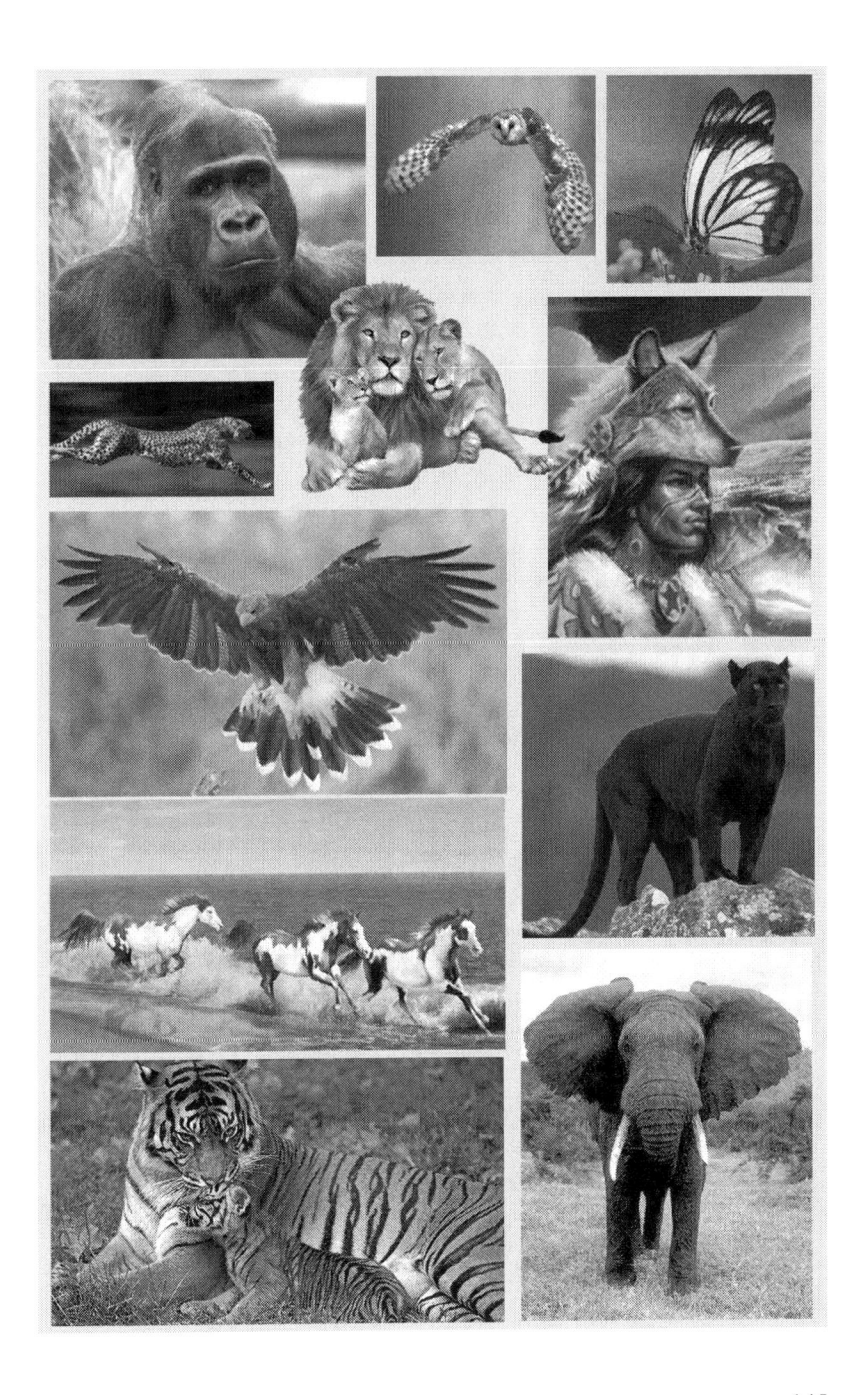

9. Guided Imagery

9.1 What is Guided Imagery?

Guided imagery is a program of directed thoughts and suggestions that guide your imagination toward a relaxed, focused state. You can use an instructor, tapes, or scripts to help you through this process.

Guided imagery is based on the concept that your body and mind are connected. Using all of your senses, your body seems to respond as though what you are imagining is real. An example often used is to imagine an orange or a lemon in great detail-the smell, the colour, the texture of the peel. Continue to imagine the smell of the lemon, and then see yourself taking a bite of the lemon and feel the juice squirting into your mouth. Many people salivate when they do this. This exercise demonstrates how your body can respond to what you are imagining.

9.2 Guided Imagery Related to Stress Management

When she needs relief from the grind of delivering major proposals, Dana Marlowe, 33, of Washington, D.C., makes some noise. "I cruise right into my toddler's playroom, and I just jam out with his toys -- the xylophone, the baby piano. I almost have 'Twinkle, Twinkle, Little Star' down," says Marlowe, a technology accessibility consultant. This kind of casual music-making can short-circuit the stress response, research shows, and keep it from becoming chronic. Stress starts in the brain and then...

You can achieve a relaxed state when you imagine all the details of a safe, comfortable place, such as a beach or a garden. This relaxed state may aid healing, learning, creativity, and performance. It may help you feel more in control of your emotions and thought processes, which may improve your attitude, health, and sense of well-being.

9.3 What is guided imagery used for?

Guided imagery has many uses. You can use it to promote relaxation, which can lower blood pressure and reduce other problems related to stress. You can also use it to help reach goals (such as losing weight or quitting smoking), manage pain, and promote healing. Using guided imagery can even help you to prepare for an athletic event or for public speaking.

9.4 Is guided imagery safe?

Guided imagery is safe. No known risks are associated with it. Guided imagery is most effective when the person teaching it has training in guided imagery techniques.

Always tell your doctor if you are using an alternative therapy or if you are thinking about combining an alternative therapy with your conventional medical treatment. It may not be safe to forgo your conventional medical treatment and rely only on an alternative therapy.

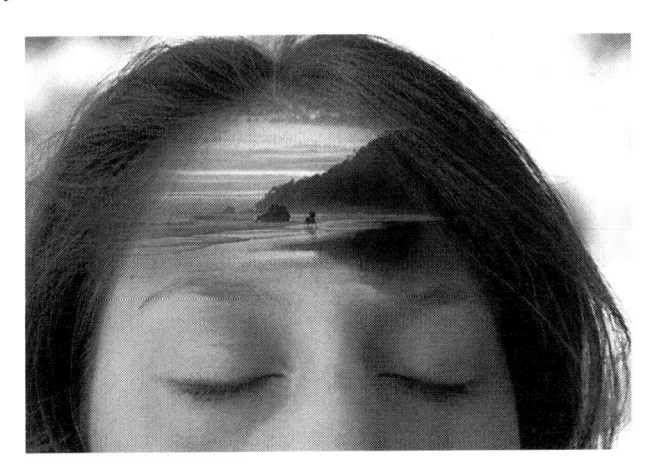

9.5 Example of a Free Relaxation Script

Relaxation to Deal with Anger

This guided relaxation script describes how to deal with anger quickly and effectively in the moment. Guides you in controlling anger and managing anger when it arises.

It's time to take a break.... and relax.... to deal with anger in a healthy, productive way.

Anger is a normal and natural emotion, and there is nothing wrong with having feelings - you are human, after all. You have the power to decide how to deal with this emotion you are experiencing.

Anger management does not mean holding anger in. It does not mean that you will never feel angry. Anger management is managing the behavioural responses that can arise when you are feeling angry.

All you really need to do right now is take a few moments just to relax, for you, to help you feel relaxed and calm. It feels good to relax. After this short relaxation session is over, you can proceed with your day, and react in a way that you choose.... relaxing for a moment now will help you to react calmly, rather than acting out of emotion.

It's okay to be angry. Just allow yourself to feel however it is you are feeling right now, noticing this feeling, but not reacting just yet. All you're doing is observing. Emotions are neither right nor wrong... they just are.

Take a deep breath in. Hold for a moment, and now breathe out.

Breathe in... hold that tension.... and now breathe out.... feeling the tension release with your breath.

Breathe in.... and out.......

in..... out.....

Keep breathing like this, slowly.... deeply.... and let your body relax a little.

Turn your attention again to how you are feeling. Notice the physical sensation of anger. Where in your body is the anger stored? Some people notice that they tighten their shoulders when they are feeling angry. Others who deal with anger notice clenched fists or tight jaws. Anger may be experienced as a feeling in the stomach.... the neck.... any one or a number of places in the body demonstrate physical symptoms of anger.

Many of these physical symptoms are uncomfortable. Some of these symptoms can be relieved right now, if you like, by relaxing your muscles. Let's relax a few areas to begin this process to deal with anger by relaxing your muscles.

Starting with your hands and arms, first tighten your hands into fists. Feel the tension in your hands and arms. Hold.... tighter.... tighter.... and relax. Let go, allowing your hands and arms to be relaxed, loose, and limp. Notice the difference between tension and relaxation.

Now see if you can create a feeling of relaxation in your shoulders. Take a moment to relax your shoulders now. You may choose to tighten the muscles, and then relax, or you can simply relax your shoulders without tensing them first. Do whatever seems to work the best.

Focus now on your face and jaws. Relax your face and jaws, tensing first if you want to. Let all the tension leave your face..... let the tension leave your jaws.... leaving your face and jaws limp, smooth, and relaxed.

Scan your body now, for remaining areas of tension. Relax each area that feels tense.... scan your body from head to toe.... relaxing each part of your body.

(pause)

Take note of how you are feeling now. Physically. Emotionally.

You are controlling anger right now, just by the fact that you have not yet reacted with angry behaviours. You have chosen to relax, to deal with anger in a healthy way.

To increase the control you have over anger, you may want to repeat some affirmations to help create realistic, rational thinking.... also called self-control thoughts.

Here are 5 affirmations for anger management to help deal with anger:

I acknowledge that I am feeling angry right now, and accept the way I feel.

I have the power to control my reactions.

I can fully experience this anger, yet wait before I take action.

I can feel angry, but calm and in control at the same time.

It's okay to feel angry.

Notice again how you are feeling. Physically, how are you feeling? Let your body relax a little more... relaxing any tense areas.

Emotionally, how are you feeling? See how emotions come and go.... anger can come and go.... it will not last forever. There is a limited time where you exercise self-control, before the anger is no longer an issue.

You may feel less angry... just as angry... or more angry now than you were at the beginning of this relaxation session.

To deal with anger that may remain, you may need a way to express the anger and get it out. You do not have to keep your emotions inside... you can choose how to express them.

You can let anger out by breathing deeply.... breathing in relaxation, and breathing out anger.... letting anger go with each breath.

There are other ways to express anger, too. You can do any of these activities after this script to allow yourself freedom to express the anger you experienced. Physical exercise, journaling, talking to someone you trust.... there are many ways to express yourself.

After the anger has decreased and you are feeling calm, you might want to address the situation that was upsetting by taking action to change the situation, or speaking to the person you were upset with. Or you may just choose to let the situation go.

Once your anger has decreased you can choose whatever option seems best. You have the right to feel a range of emotions, including anger, and to express these emotions in healthy ways that you choose.

I'll conclude this script with some breathing.

Take a deep breath in.... and out.....

in..... out.... relaxing with each breath

in..... out....

in..... out....

Keep breathing deeply to deal with anger and feel relaxed and calm.

Congratulate yourself for dealing with anger with relaxation.

I'll count now from 5 to 1. Imagine that right now, you are at a 5, and that when I reach 1 you will be feeling awake and alert, yet calm, peaceful, and relaxed.

5 – 4 – 3 – 2 – 1

Sources:

http://www.webmd.com/balance/stress-management/tc/guided-imagery-topic-overview

Source: http://www.innerhealthstudio.com/deal-with-anger.html

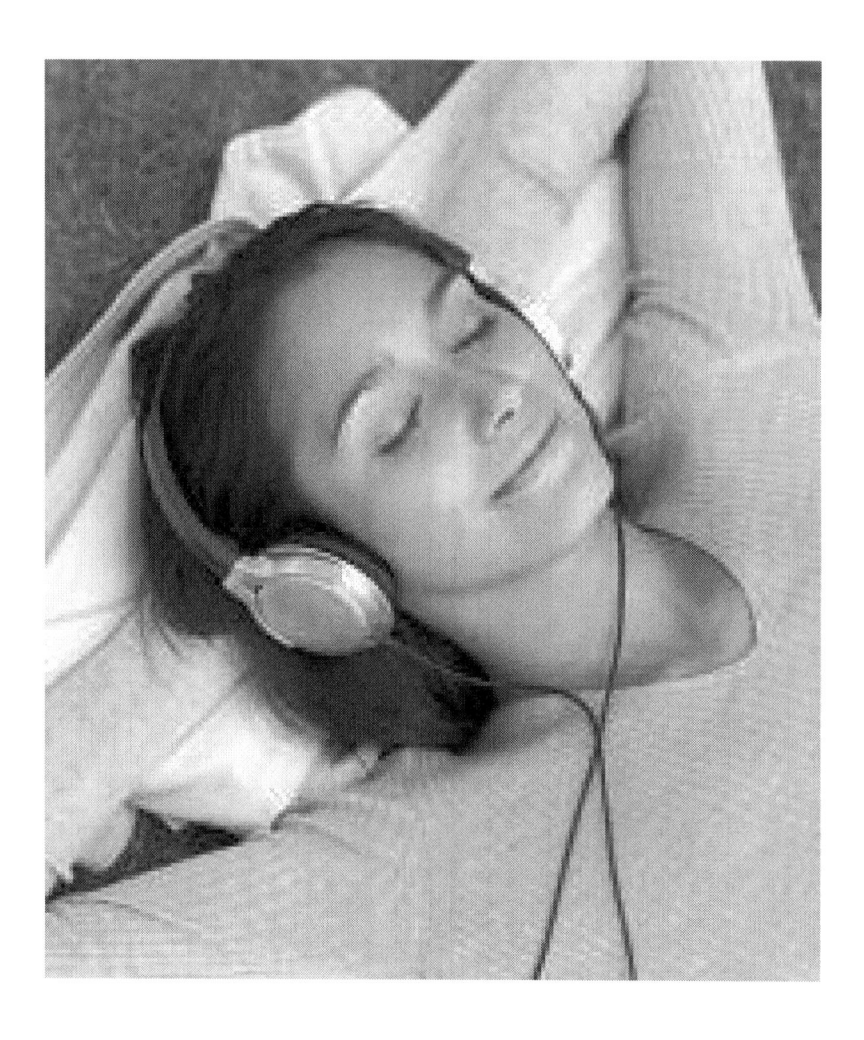

10. The Power of the Mind's Eye

10.1 See without seeing

Our ability to see is literal and figurative, in that our brains can generate images regardless of whether or not we are physically seeing an object with our eyes. The ability to "see" without seeing, known as mental imagery, can be used as a way to improve athletic performance, to instil positive thinking, and to treat the symptoms of certain mental conditions. For example, the use of meditation to focus the mind on a single object can reduce the occurrence of intrusive thoughts in conditions such as OCD (1) and ADHD. Though our general understanding of the ways in which mental imagery can affect us is pretty good, how and why we use it remain unanswered questions.

Knowing how the eye works and how we physiologically process visual information has brought to light some of the details concerning the underlying physical basis of mental imagery. At the back of the eye lies a thin, delicate layer of cells sensitive to light. Light waves detected by these cells are converted into electrical signals that pulse along neurons extending from the back of the eye to an area of the brain involved in visual information processing. Light waves flow into electrical signals flow into meaningful images. This gives us our sense of vision.

It is no secret that the images generated by the brain extend to the human conscious. Images originating in the brain are manifested as responses, emotional or otherwise, that are a result of activity in the matching mind. This enables us not only to see but also to react to what we see. In the case of particularly moving or evocative images, these reactions, positive or negative, are often stronger than reactions elicited by words describing the images.

But visualization, in a philosophical sense, is larger than the ability to see. With the exception of people who are born blind, the brain can generate images in the absence of visual input. In the mind, this ability is translated into the reproduction of pictures of life, of our worlds, that can affect us in profound ways. This phenomenon was recognized by philosophers and scientists centuries ago.

Aristotle identified phantasia, what has since been interpreted as imagination. However, Aristotle's use of the term phantasia appears to be more closely associated with what humans actively perceive, or see. This realization, and the later assumption that an object being physically seen cannot be imagined at the same moment, conflicts with the equation of phantasia to imagination. Beyond this, Plato adapted phantasia to describe perception, using phainesthai, meaning "to appear," in relation to mental processes. However, today, phantasia remains understood as fictional imagery, or fantasy. The modern term that essentially describes Aristotle's and Plato's concepts is mental imagery, forming an image of something in our minds in the absence of seeing that something.

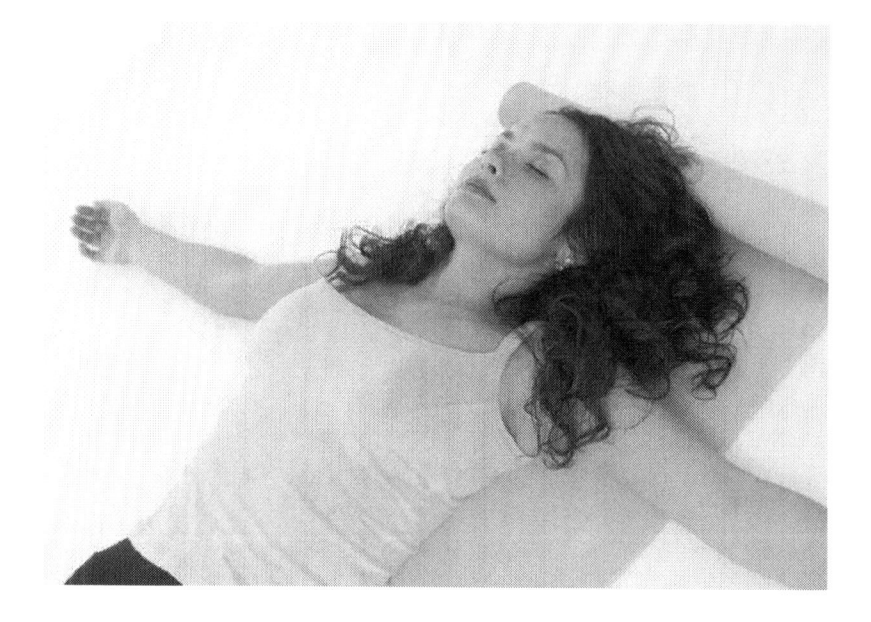

Mental imagery is easily confused with hallucination, because the two share superficial similarities. However, mental imagery differs from hallucination in that we have control over the images we generate. Our eyes accept visual input of all kinds from the world around us, but our brains and minds are capable of focusing on single images, images that we have the power to select.

Today there still is no clear association connecting what we see with what we recreate in our minds and how we respond. But perhaps our ability to select our minds' images explains why what we see and what we "see" are sometimes two very different things.

(1) OCD: obsessive-compulsive disorder, also called obsessive-compulsive neurosis, type of mental disorder in which an individual experiences obsessions or compulsions or both. Either the obsessive thought or the compulsive act may occur singly, or both may appear in sequence.

(2) ADHD: attention-deficit/hyperactivity disorder, a behavioral syndrome characterized by inattention and distractibility, restlessness, inability to sit still, and difficulty concentrating on one thing for any period of time. ADHD most commonly occurs in children, though an increasing number of adults are being diagnosed with the disorder. ADHD is three times more common in males than in females and occurs in approximately 3 to 6 percent of all children. Although behaviours characteristic of the syndrome are evident in all cultures, they have garnered the most attention in the United States, where ADHD is the most commonly diagnosed childhood psychiatric disorder.

Source:

Encyclopaedia Britannica Blog - Kara Rogers

http://www.britannica.com/blogs/2008/09/mental-imagery-the-power-of-the-minds-eye/

10.2 Eyes Wide Shut: seeing with closed eyes

A mental image is an experience that, on most occasions, significantly resembles the experience of perceiving some object, event, or scene, but occurs when the relevant object, event, or scene is not actually present to the senses. There are sometimes episodes, particularly on falling asleep (hypnagogic imagery) and waking up (hypnopompic), when the mental imagery, being of a rapid, phantasmagoric and involuntary character, defies perception, presenting a kaleidoscopic field, in which no distinct object can be discerned.

The nature of these experiences, what makes them possible, and their function (if any) have long been subjects of research and controversy in philosophy, psychology, cognitive science, and more recently, neuroscience. As contemporary researchers use the expression, mental images (or mental imagery) can occur in the form of any sense, so that we may experience auditory images, olfactory images, and so forth. However, the vast majority of philosophical and scientific investigations of the topic focus upon visual mental imagery. It has been assumed that, like humans, many types of animals are capable of experiencing mental images. Due to the fundamentally subjective nature of the phenomenon, there is little to no evidence either for or against this view.

Philosophers such as George Berkeley and David Hume, and early experimental psychologists such as Wilhelm Wundt and William James, understood ideas in general to be mental images, and today it is very widely believed that much imagery functions as mental representations (or mental models), playing an important role in memory and thinking. Some have gone so far as to suggest that images are best understood to be, by definition, a form of inner, mental or neural representation; in the case of hypnagogic and hypnapompic imagery, it is not representational at all. Others reject the view that the image experience may be identical with (or directly caused by) any such representation in the mind or the brain, but do not take account of the non-representational forms of imagery.

In 2010 IBM applied for a patent on how to extract mental images of human faces from the human brain. It uses a feedback loop based on brain measurements of the fusiform face area in the brain which activates proportionate with degree of facial recognition.

10.3 How mental images form in the brain

Common examples of mental images include daydreaming and the mental visualization that occurs while reading a book. When a musician hears a song, he or she can sometimes "see" the song notes in their head, as well as hear them with all their tonal qualities. This is considered different from an after-effect, such as an after-image. Calling up an image in our minds can be a voluntary act, so it can be characterized as being under various degrees of conscious control.

According to psychologist and cognitive scientist Steven Pinker, our experiences of the world are represented in our minds as mental images. These mental images can then be associated and compared with others, and can be used to synthesize completely new images. In this view, mental images allow us to form useful theories of how the world works by formulating likely sequences of mental images in our heads without having to directly experience that outcome. Whether other creatures have this capability is debatable.

10.4 Mental representation

Mental images are an important topic in classical and modern philosophy, as they are central to the study of knowledge. In the Republic, book VII, Plato uses the metaphor of a prisoner in a cave, bound and unable to move, sitting with his back to a fire and watching the shadows cast on the wall in front of him by people carrying objects behind his back. The objects that they are carrying are representations of real things in the world. The prisoner, explains

Socrates, is like a human being making mental images from the sense data that he experiences.

More recently, Bishop George Berkeley has proposed similar ideas in his theory of idealism. Berkeley stated that reality is equivalent to mental images — our mental images are not a copy of another material reality, but that reality itself. Berkeley, however, sharply distinguished between the images that he considered to constitute the external world, and the images of individual imagination. According to Berkeley, only the latter are considered "mental imagery" in the contemporary sense of the term.

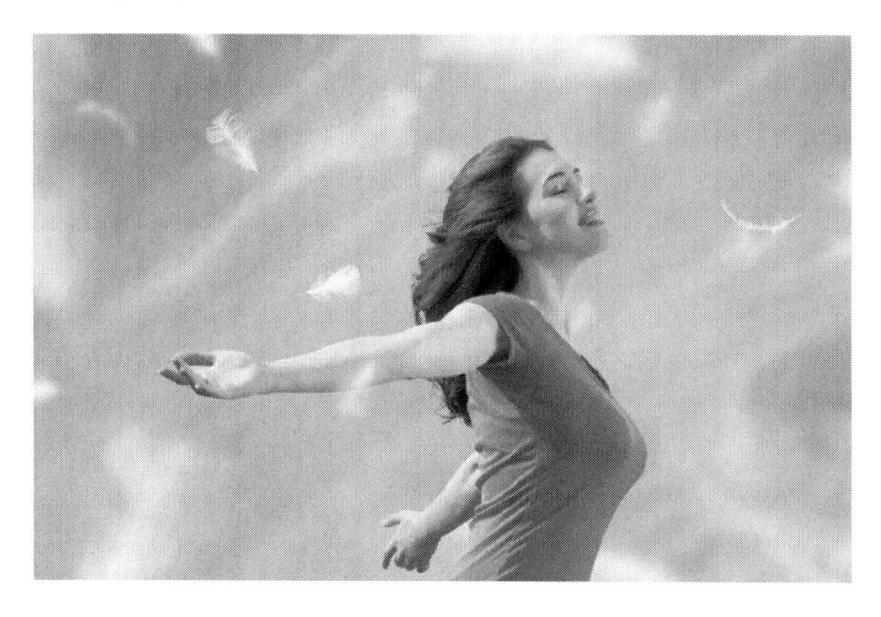

David Deutsch addresses Johnson's objection to idealism in The Fabric of Reality when he states that if we judge the value of our mental images of the world by the quality and quantity of the sense data that they can explain, then the most valuable mental image — or theory — that we currently have is that the world has a real independent existence and that humans have successfully evolved by building up and adapting patterns of mental images to explain it. This is an important idea in scientific thought.[why?]

Critics of scientific realism ask how the inner perception of mental images actually occurs. This is sometimes called the "homunculus problem" (see also the mind's eye). The problem is similar to asking how the images you see on a computer screen exist in the memory of the computer. To scientific materialism, mental images and the perception of them must be brain-states. According to critics,[who?] scientific realists cannot explain where the images and their perceiver exist in the brain. To use the analogy of the computer screen, these critics argue that cognitive science and psychology has been unsuccessful in identifying either the component in the brain (i.e. "hardware") or the mental processes that store these images (i.e. "software").

10.5 Mental imagery in experimental psychology

Cognitive psychologists and (later) cognitive neuroscientists have empirically tested some of the philosophical questions related to whether and how the human brain uses mental imagery in cognition.

One theory of the mind that was examined in these experiments was the "brain as serial computer" philosophical metaphor of the 1970s. Psychologist Zenon Pylyshyn theorized that the human mind processes mental images by decomposing them into an underlying mathematical proposition. Roger Shepard and Jacqueline Metzler challenged that view by presenting subjects with 2D line drawings of groups of 3D block "objects" and asking them to determine whether that "object" was the same as a second figure, some of which were rotations of the first "object". Shepard and Metzler proposed that if we decomposed and then mentally re-imaged the objects into basic mathematical propositions, as the then-dominant view of cognition "as a serial digital computer" assumed, then it would be expected that the time it took to determine whether the object was the same or not would be independent of how much the object was rotated.

Shepard and Metzler found the opposite: a linear relationship between the degree of rotation in the mental imagery task and the time it took participants to reach their answer.

This mental rotation finding implied that the human mind — and the human brain — maintains and manipulates mental images as topographic and topological wholes, an implication that was quickly put to test by psychologists. Stephen Kosslyn and colleagues showed in a series of neuroimaging experiments that the mental image of objects like the letter "F" are mapped, maintained and rotated as an image-like whole in areas of the human visual cortex. Moreover, Kosslyn's work showed that there were considerable similarities between the neural mappings for imagined stimuli and perceived stimuli. The authors of these studies concluded that while the neural processes they studied rely on mathematical and computational underpinnings, the brain also seems optimized to handle the sort of mathematics that constantly computes a series of topologically-based images rather than calculating a mathematical model of an object.

Recent studies in neurology and neuropsychology on mental imagery have further questioned the "mind as serial computer" theory, arguing instead that human mental imagery manifests both visually and kinesthetically. For example, several studies have provided evidence that people are slower at rotating line drawings of objects such as hands in directions incompatible with the joints of the human body, and that patients with painful, injured arms are slower at mentally rotating line drawings of the hand from the side of the injured arm.

Some psychologists, including Kosslyn, have argued that such results occur because of interference in the brain between distinct systems in the brain that process the visual and motor mental imagery. Subsequent neuroimaging studies showed that the interference between the motor and visual imagery system could be induced by having participants physically handle actual 3D blocks glued together to form objects similar to those depicted in the line-drawings. Amorim et al. have recently shown that when a cylindrical "head" was added to Shepard and Metzler's line drawings of 3D block figures, participants were quicker and more accurate at solving mental rotation problems. They argue that motoric embodiment is not just "interference" that inhibits visual mental imagery, but is capable of facilitating mental imagery.

These and numerous related studies have led to a relative consensus within cognitive science, psychology, neuroscience and philosophy on the neural status of mental images. Researchers generally agree that while there is no homunculus inside the head viewing these mental images, our brains do form and maintain mental images as image-like wholes. The problem of exactly how these images are stored and manipulated within the human brain, particularly within language and communication, remains a fertile area of study.

One of the longest running research topics on the mental image has been the fact that people report large individual differences in the vividness of their images. Special questionnaires have been developed to assess such differences, including the Vividness of Visual Imagery Questionnaire (VVIQ) developed by David Marks. Laboratory studies have suggested that the subjectively reported variations in imagery vividness are associated with different neural states within the brain and also different cognitive competences such as the ability to accurately recall information presented in pictures Rodway, Gillies and Schepman used a novel long-term change detection task to determine whether participants with low and high vividness scores on the VVIQ2 showed any performance differences. Rodway et al. found that high vividness participants were significantly more accurate at detecting salient changes to pictures compared to low vividness participants. This replicated an earlier study.

Recent studies have found that individual differences in VVIQ scores can be used to predict changes in a person's brain while visualizing different activities. Functional magnetic resonance imaging (fMRI) was used to study the association between early visual cortex activity relative to the whole brain while participants visualized themselves or another person bench pressing or stair climbing. Reported image vividness correlates significantly with the relative fMRI signal in the visual cortex. Thus individual differences in the vividness of visual imagery can be measured objectively.

Logie, Pernet, Buonocore and Della Sala (2011) used behavioural and fMRI data for mental rotation from individuals reporting vivid and poor imagery on the VVIQ. Groups differed in in brain activation patterns suggesting that the groups performed the same tasks in different ways. These findings help to explain the lack of association previously reported between VVIQ scores and mental rotation performance.

10.6 Training and learning styles

Some educational theorists have drawn from the idea of mental imagery in their studies of learning styles. Proponents of these theories state that people often have learning processes which emphasize visual, auditory, and kinesthetic systems of experience.[citation needed] According to these theorists, teaching in multiple overlapping sensory systems benefits learning, and they encourage teachers to use content and media that integrates well with the visual, auditory, and kinesthetic systems whenever possible.

Educational researchers have examined whether the experience of mental imagery affects the degree of learning. For example, imagining playing a 5-finger piano exercise (mental practice) resulted in a significant improvement in performance over no mental practice — though not as significant as that produced by physical practice. The authors of the study stated that "mental practice alone seems to be sufficient to promote the modulation of neural circuits involved in the early stages of motor skill learning."

10.7 The Himalayan traditions

Vajrayana Buddhism, Bön and Tantra in general, utilize sophisticated visualization or imaginal (in the language of Jean Houston of Transpersonal Psychology) processes in the thoughtform construction of the yidam sadhana, kye-rim, and dzog-rim modes of meditation and in the yantra, thangka, and mandala traditions, where holding the fully realized form in the mind is a prerequisite prior to creating an 'authentic' new art work that will provide a sacred support or foundation for deity.

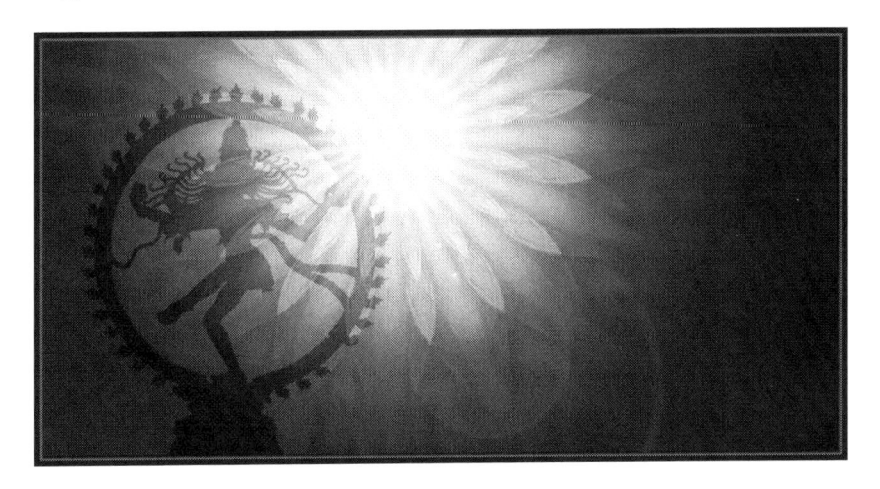

Source:

From Wikipedia, the free encyclopedia
Text is available under the Creative Commons Attribution-ShareAlike License; additional terms may apply. By using this site, you agree to the Terms of Use and Privacy Policy.
Wikipedia® is a registered trademark of the Wikimedia Foundation, Inc., a non-profit organization.

11. Healing Power and Visualization

From Kathryn C. Shafer, Ph.D.

Mental imagery, sometimes called visualization, guided imagery, and often used interchangeably with the practice of meditation and hypnosis, is the language used by the mind to communicate and make sense about the inner and outer worlds (Shafer & Greenfield, 2000).

Imagery, refers to the awareness of sensory (physical), and perceptual (cognitive), experiences which have been used in a variety of health and healing practices in the Western world for over three decades (Heinschel, 2002). Meditation, mindfulness, hypnosis, and yoga are also techniques commonly used in Behavioral Health Programs today to assist in high-level awareness health education sessions (Kabot-Zinn,1990).

While there is something unique and peculiar about thinking in mental images, or understanding the meaning of "pictures in the head" as it applies to health and well being, this uniqueness is to receiving attention in the theoretical and research literature (Pslyshyn, 2002).

Given the diverse role of the imagination appears to have in healing, the difficulty in studying the invisible world scientifically, religious groups who oppose such practices, and the differences in preconceptions held by practitioners, it is no surprise that there are many distinct views on the practice and value of mental imagery (Pinker & Kosslyn, 1983, Snaith, 1998).

11.1 Role of Imagination in Healing

In the last decade, interest in the practice of mental imagery, and the role of the imagination in health and well being, has dramatically increased as a popular approach for treating a wide variety of psychiatric, medical concerns, and enhancing sports performance (Shafer & Greenfield, 2002; Bloom, 1998; Epstein, 1989). In fact, ten million North Americans of all ages admit openly to practicing some form of imagery or meditation, to reduce stress, boost the immune system, and cope with life threatening illnesses. This number has doubled compared to admitted devotees a decade ago (Stein, 2003; O'Donnell, Maurice, & Beattie, 2002). While the principles of mental imagery have been utilized in healing since the beginning of medical history, recent pioneers embracing the scientific merit of mental imagery are transforming the healing practices in Western medicine (Ader, 1981; LeShan, 1989; Selye, 1956; Simonton & Henson, 1992; Borysenko, 1988; Benson, 1975; Brigham, 1994).

11.2 Mental States and Physical Health

Mental States and Physical Health Are Intimately Connected. The era of health care reform has placed a great emphasis on brief therapies, behaviorial health, and alternative practices involving the cooperative relationship of the therapist, and the active participation of the client (Elliott, 2003). As a result, doctors, health care providers, therapists, and patients acknowledge that mental states and physical health are intimately connected (Lemonick, 2003). Advances and shifts in health care practice have stimulated education, training, and the clinical application of imagery for the treatment of mental health, substance abuse, and medical problems. Mainstream Americans no longer have to search for gurus in the mountains or the Far East to inquire about the practice of mental imagery. Information is now offered and training provided in schools, hospitals, law firms, government buildings, corporate offices, and prisons (Gruzelier, 2002; Stein, 2003).

The central theme that emerges from empirical research is the impact of the client's sensory experience during the imaginal process

(Heinschel, 2002). Clients do not have something "done" to them, they live an actual experience during the imagery exercise using the practitioner (clinician, health care worker, as the guide). While the eyes are either open (focused on a point in front of them) or closed, the client is guided through the exercise in the clinical setting (office, hospital, home, etc.), to be practiced as "prescribed" (i.e. x times daily) on their own between sessions (one time only, daily for seven days, or for twenty one days) depending on the presenting problem and the individual (Shafer & Greenfield, 2002).

11.3 Case Studies

The following case examples illustrate how mental imagery can be utilized in a variety of health concerns:

Case Example #1

Sandra, a 43-year-old attorney, has been asthmatic since childhood. Despite using a variety of approaches, she has always felt enslaved to her disease. She has tried both ignoring her condition and catering to it. Though everything seems to help for a time, nothing gives her the release she seeks. She is tired of searching for a solution which constantly evades her. Feeling drained and confused, she seeks out a clinician trained in the use of mental imagery as a treatment of last resort.

The therapist asks Sandra to close her eyes, turns her senses inward, and does some reverse breathing (exhaling first though her mouth, then inhaling through her nose). With this simple preparation, Sandra enters the world of her imagination where anything is possible – for here there are no rules, no diagnoses or prognoses, in fact, no limitations of any kind. Using an imagery exercise called "Liberation From Slavery," Sandra sees and feels herself chained to her illness which appears to her as a large beast pressing her down, its foot planted firmly on her chest. Uncomfortable as this image may be, once she sees it she has the opportunity to acknowledge it (in effect to experience it), and to make a change. Using her imagination, she finds a key that unlocks the chains, breaks free of the beast, and releases herself from its power. Suddenly, the beast begins shrinking, while Sandra grows taller. As the chains fall away, the restriction and heaviness in her chest diminish. She feels lighter, her breathing becomes easier, and the sense of fear and powerlessness she had been feeling is replaced by hope and clarity.

When the imagery exercise is completed, the clinician as the guide, instructs her to breathe out and open her eyes. At this time, the therapist asks Sandra how she feels, and asks Sandra to describe her experience from the exercise in the present tense. She is encouraged to try this exercise (the prescribed dose), every day for at least seven days, up to 21 days, and to record her experiences (including night dreams) until her next appointment.

The benefits Sandra derives from doing this exercise are far reaching and immediate. Her imagery acts as a mirror that reveals her from the inside out. Instantaneously, from the imagery exercise she has learned truths about herself that until now she has overlooked, even denied. Indeed, she is stronger, "taller," more powerful than she ever suspected. By freeing herself from the chains (which she sensed were her beliefs and fears about her illness), she becomes bigger than this disease, something she had always felt was all powerful, too much for her to handle. In changing the image, which she does by using the key to release herself, she has affected her beliefs, thoughts, and feelings in a positive, and liberating way. In doing this, she has gone beyond ordinary thinking where such things are "impossible," and has become her own authority, the one who is ultimately in control of her choices in life (Shafer & Greenfield, 2002).

Case Example # 2

Dee is a 55 year old nurse who works many hours and is the sole supporter of her family. She presents at the office with her arms scarred and scabbed severely from her digging and scratching. After discussing the various issues in her life that are "making her itch", she is guided through a mental imagery exercise (Epstein, 1989) for general relaxation. Several days later, Dee emails the clinician the following (personal communication, with Shafer, 2003) exercise she developed on her own, evolving from the general relaxation exercise she was given in session. Her intention is to stop the itching and heal the wounds on her arms:

I sit in a quiet place (if at all possible). I close my eyes gently and take a few deep breaths. During this time, my mind travels to the spleen and watches as red blood cells (rbcs) come out to travel around the body. They travel to the heart and to the lungs and I watch as they pick up oxygen and return to the heart to be sent to all parts of the body. At this time, the rbcs have also picked up glucose and there are white blood cells and antibodies travelling with them. I view them as they descend through the network of arteries, arterioles, and capillaries and then, they are at the sites that need healing. I like to visualize the right and left sides separately, but if I am tired and start fighting sleep, then I pull my perspective back and watch both sides at the same time. I see the rbcs leaving oxygen and glucose at the base of the lesions. I see the antibodies surrounding the areas to prevent infection and I see the wbcs backing up the antibodies.

I then pull my perspective back and gently stroke each arm separately and visualize more blood going to the areas to help them heal. The last thing I do is to take several deep breaths and tell my body that I do not want it to show me evidence of my anger, frustration, or stress. I tell it that there is no need for my body to hurt itself. Then I take three long breaths out and with each exhale I say (imaginally): "With this breath, I breathe out all of my anger, with this breath, I breathe out all of my stress, with this breath I breath out all my frustration."

Like Sandra, the impact for Dee was immediate. She stopped itching within the week, created her own imagery exercise making her the authority over her healing, and the scabs were healed (without scarring) within one month. The confidence and esteem Dee gained from the creation of her own exercise and the results she achieved from doing the work herself drastically improved her sense of self. Clients gain a sense of mastery and call recall such achievements when future health challenges present senses of doubt, and helplessness.

11.4 Summary

As with the beginning of all habits, start with simple relaxation exercises first, perhaps with yourself and other colleagues to gain comfort and familiarity with engaging the imagination and each of the five senses. The mind and the body can interact in many ways to bring about health and illness as is introduced throughout this chapter. At first these interactions may be difficult to understand or see, however practice observing and reading the images provided in the exercises with a deeper appreciation. Experiment with all the possible ways to gain access to the sensory world of the client. For example start listening in a more active way such as listening to music. Or, if the client has trouble imaging, involve the sense of smell or taste or touch, integrate aromatherapy in the practice. Clients may like to write impressions from the work in a journal, record dreams, and utilize the therapist as the teacher or guide in their journey.

What may be discovered as the work of mental imagery continues, is that this not only attunes the therapist's ability to image, but how to expand in this work with clients. While research is a challenge and is highly debated in this work, the evidence based research must continue to further the credibility of this mind body practice.

11.5 Wellness and Wholeness Visualizations

Visualization helps no matter what your challenges are or how wonderful your current situation is. Visualization can be a powerful tool for improvement as well as for maintaining a happy life style. Wellness imagery can help you turn any negatives into positives. Beautiful pictures can reinforce the perfect life you are living or hope to begin living. Choose images that represent good health, fitness, and happiness. Whatever represents your ideal of "love" or "perfection" or "tranquility" those are the pictures you want to focus on.

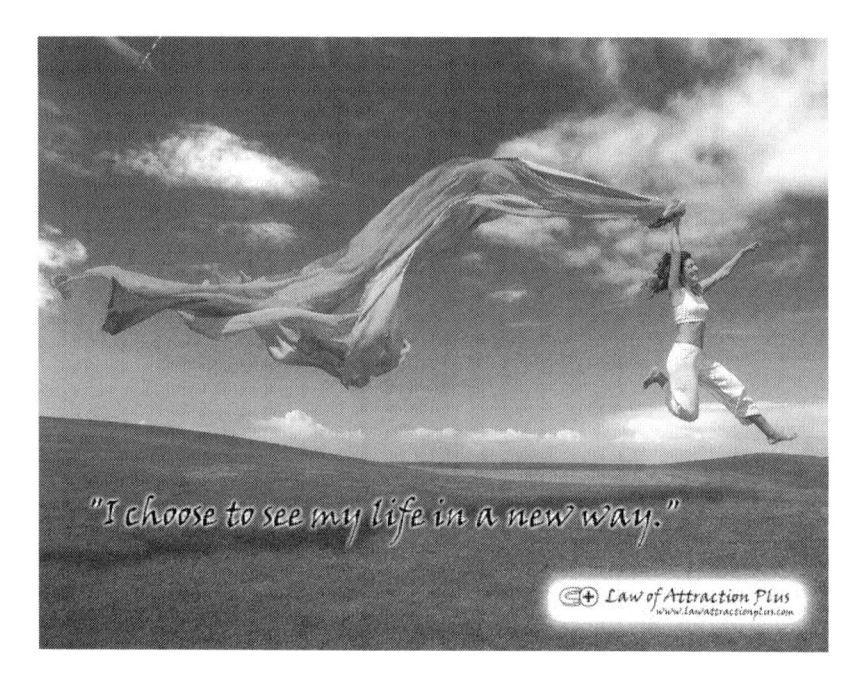

"I choose to see my life in a new way."

Law of Attraction Plus
www.lawofattractionplus.com

Sources:

Http://healing.about.com/od/visualization/a/imagery_shafer.htm

http://healing.about.com/od/visualization/a/powerofmind.htm
http://drmiller.com/learning-center/healyourself/

11.6 The Healing Power of the Mind

From Linda Mackenzie

A picture is worth a thousand words.

We have heard that saying before. This phrase is certainly true in the case of visualization. Visualization, a form of self-hypnosis, is a tool anyone can use to help foster healing. By providing positive pictures (creative imagery) and self-suggestion, visualization can change emotions that subsequently have a physical effect on the body.

Our belief system is based upon the accumulation of verbal and non-verbal suggestions that have been gathered throughout our life experience. Through patterns of repetition and its associated rewards and punishment we learn to create our own perception of reality. In essence, we therefore become what we think. In healing, repetitive use of positive visualization allows access to the mind-body connection. This lets the mind and body work together to foster the healing process of the body on a physical level. What is the mind-body connection and how does it work? When we have an emotion it generates a feeling that turns into a physical sensation.

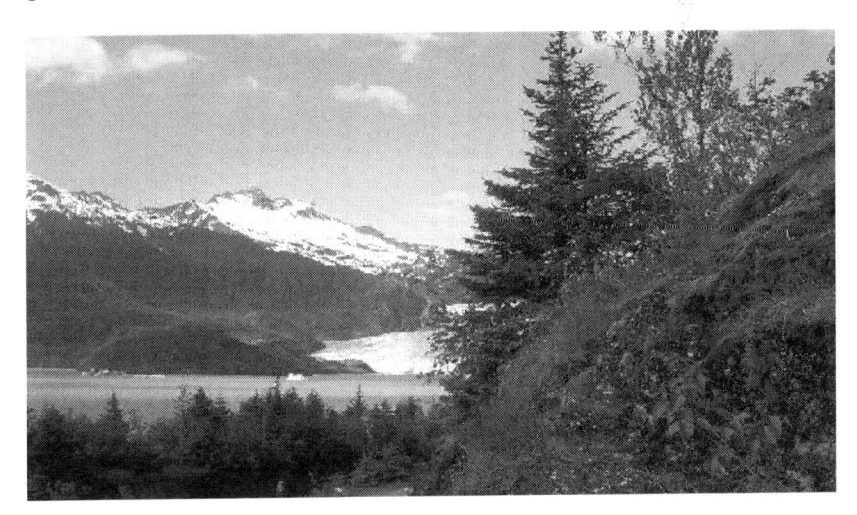

For example: You are watching a horror movie, you feel frightened and then get a chill up your spine. In this case you were getting a negative suggestion through your sensory perception (sight and sound), that produced an emotion of fear which turned into the physical sensation of chills up your spine. Visualization uses positive images to produce positive emotions that manifest into positive physical sensations in the body.

Sounds simple, but does it work? Can what we think actually have an effect on healing? Bodies do react to the thoughts you make. Our psychological/emotional state affects the endocrine system. For example, the emotion of fear is related to adrenaline. If no feeling of fear exists there is no adrenaline and the same applies in reverse- no adrenaline, no fear. They work in relationship to each other. Wherever a thought goes there is a body chemical reaction.

The hypothalamus, the emotional centre of the brain, transforms emotions into physical response. The receptor of neuropeptides, the hypothalamus also controls the bodyís appetite, blood sugar levels, body temperature, adrenal and pituitary glands, heart, lung, digestive and circulatory systems. Neuropeptides, the chemical messenger hormones, carry emotions back and forth between the mind and body. They link perception in the brain to the body via organs, hormones and cellular activity. Neuropeptides influence every major section of the immune system, so the body and mind do work together as one unit.

The brain is a highly efficient system that is connected to every cell in your body by billions of connections. It is divided into two sides ñ the left, logical side (words, logic, rational thought) and the right creative side (imagination and intuition). Day to day circumstances usually are met in a logical, left brain mode; however by yielding to the right, creative side of the brain we actually restore balance in the brain. This allows access to the mind-body connection to achieve what you want. The right side of the brain automatically steers you to your goal. It totally accepts what you want to accomplish without giving an opinion and acts upon it without judgement. That is why visualization targets the right, creative side of the brain and not the left, logical side.

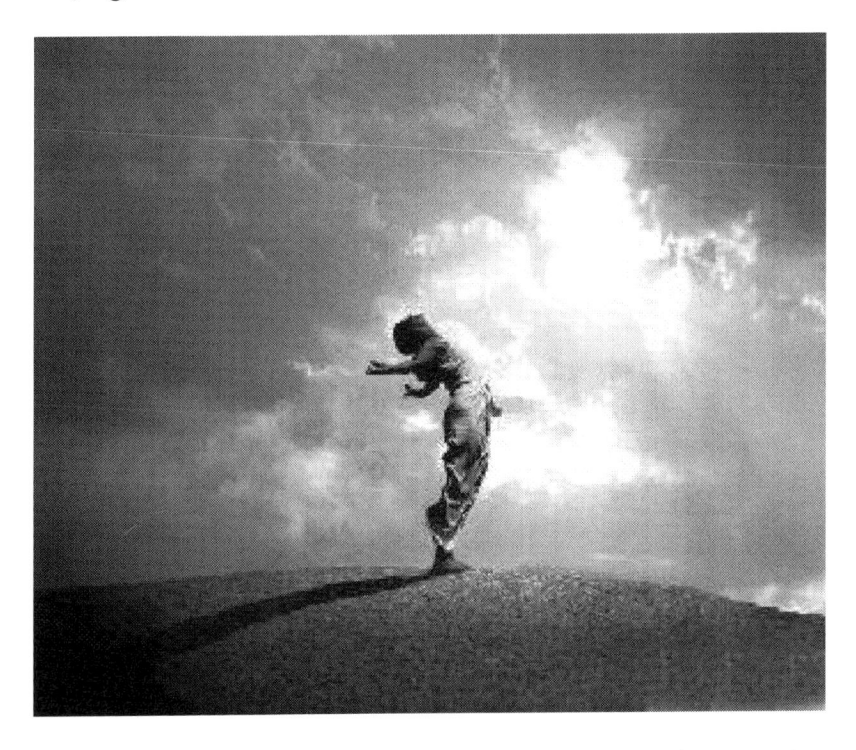

Positive thought is essential to producing positive results. Negative thoughts and emotions lower the immune system, while positive thought and emotions actually boost the immune system. To maximize success of visualization as a support to the healing process, the following suggestions are offered:

11.7 Define Your Specific Intention

Visualization puts your intention of what you want to work. The more specific the intention, the more specific the results. Remember whatever you believe is what your body will do.

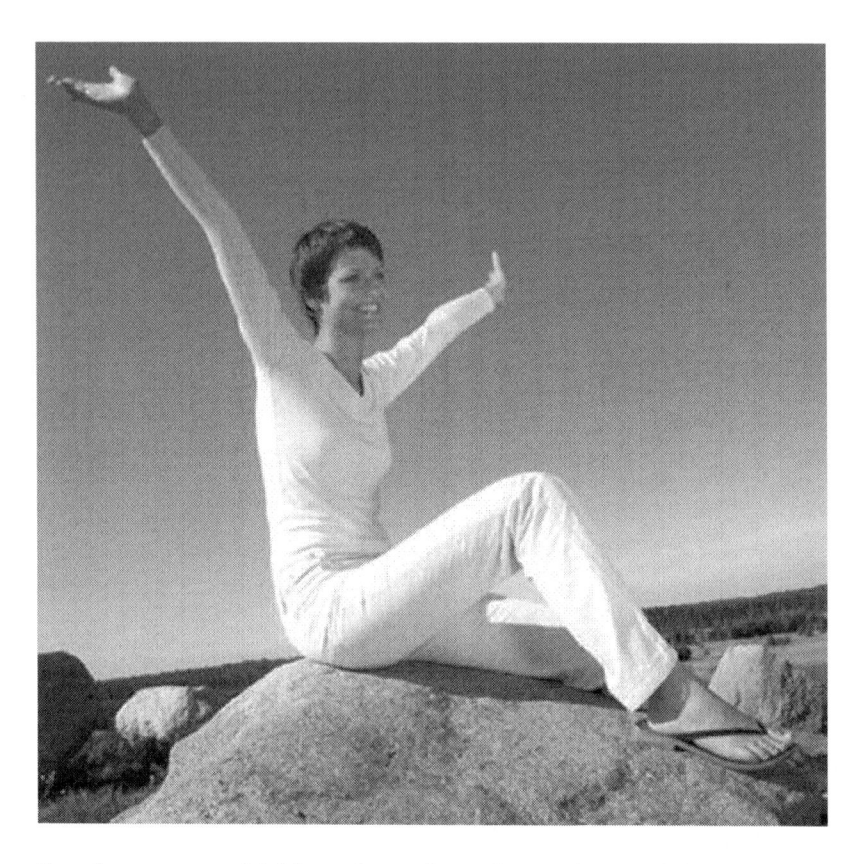

So when you are thinking of your intention make sure it is:

Clear
Specific
Achievable
You feel, know and trust it is being accomplished
Take Responsibility

Trying to do visualization without taking responsibility will prove to be futile experience. To accomplish what you want you must take action and responsibility. Visualization usually takes about 6 weeks to work. It is done once in the morning and before bedtime. Some people do see or feel results the very first time but remember everyone's body and mind are different and so is the way they process information so have patience.

Responsibility is:

- ✓ Be accountable to and for yourself
- ✓ Make a commitment
- ✓ Do visualization regularly
- ✓ Be persistent and patient
- ✓ Keep positive
- ✓ Get Mentally Relaxed

A relaxed state puts allows you direct access to your subconscious mind.

Here are some steps to help you relax:

- Find a quiet place. Relax in a favorite chair or lie down.
- Get comfortable and loosen clothing
- Uncross your arms and legs
- Get centred by focusing on the breath and breathing (this activates the vagus nerve which is the major quieting nerve in the body)
- Totally relax your body and mind
- Visualize

Once you are relaxed the next step is to actualize your visualization.

- Think of or speak your intention out loud.
- Close your eyes and imagine yourself in the healing process or as you want to be.
- Watch as your body heals you
- Feel the healing taking place
- Know the healing is being accomplished

If you have difficulty you may want to try one or more of these methods:

- Use creative imagery like seeing the cells in your body healing you; your immune system fighting off invaders; your pain being taken away by healing mud
- Imagine yourself in a very beautiful place whole, healthy and happy
- Try reading scripts from a visualization or self-hypnosis book
- Try making your own tape in your own voice

11.8 How to Heal Yourself

Visualization does work to help boost your body back to health. Don't just work on the body, add the mind to maximize your healing process with visualization.

In his blog publication "How to Heal Yourself", dr Emmett Miller, MD writes that the process to heal yourself is actually simple:

You can heal yourself! In fact, you are the only one who can.

The right food, the right exercise, the right medications, the right relationships -all these can help support your healing process, but not unless you intentionally cause them to.

Your conscious, intentional mind (which is separate from, though connected to, your subconscious mind and nervous system) is the key to your self healing.

1. First you need to understand the process with your intellect, the part capable of critical thinking that realizes the value of evidence-based reasoning.

2. The next step in healing any system is that the system become aware of its identity as a system. For you this means freeing yourself

from distraction and focusing on who you are, your true values, purpose, goals, and vision.

3. Then you learn how to read the signals and messages that come from within and how to balance your system — physically, mentally, and emotionally.

To start, you relax until you reach a pleasant state of deep relaxation and meditation, bringing you into the present, emptying your mind of distractions and your body of toxins, and preparing the cells of your body to receive your self healing instructions.

Then you use mental imagery to send your healing instructions to your body and reinforce their impact

11.9 Guided Imagery.

Guided Imagery is a very valuable tool for self healing. This process involves holding specific healing imagery in the mind while in the receptive "Healing State." This results in relief of stress, and the activation of your unconscious healing and corrective processes are mobilized. In a very real sense, you are "reprogramming" your mind and rewiring your brain. Your goal is to restore internal coherence and balance, and thus to help heal your body, emotions, mind and behaviour.

Each time you repeat these experiences, you are re-scripting your body, your emotional state, and how you will respond in future situations. You will discover this is a powerful way to mentally rehearse, through guided imagery, your desired behaviours of mind and body, much as athletes or actors mentally rehearse their performances.

These new behaviours may have to do with modifying how the internal organs of your body operate, how you talk to yourself, your personal habits, how you interact with others, etc. Diet, exercise, rest, prayer, meditation, and other modalities of re-balancing the system may be needed, but all these require us to change our mental behaviour in order to apply them. Thus, the mind-body axis is always primary in healing yourself. Change Your Mind – Change Your Life.

11.10 The Six Steps of Self Healing

1. Education — Obtain as much accurate information as possible about health and healing. Learn as much about your constitution and about your condition, the symptoms, aetiology, and therapy, including the role of stress, diet, emotions and exercise. Learn about the different options for treating your condition. To begin your education consider reading about Mind-Body Medicine.

2. Relaxation — Deep Relaxation is essential for rapid healing because it is the direct antidote to stress. In addition, relaxation empties your mind of distractions, and thus allows you to self-program new, more desirable self healing behaviours — both at the visible (macroscopic) level, and in the microscopic behaviour of the cells of your body. Deep relaxation is also the key to programming mind and body for peak performance in any endeavour — sports, profession, or personal life (yes, even sexual).

3. Entering "The Healing State" — Here the mind is open to re-scripting and the body accepts new healthy images and emotions. Re-scripting is a powerful way to mentally rehearse desired behaviours of the mind and body, much as athletes or actors mentally rehearse their performances. These guided imagery & meditation CDs and .MP3 downloads will teach you to do this through simple, logical, straightforward, and highly enjoyable guided imagery experiences. The experience and your ability to use the Healing State becomes progressively more powerful with a few minutes a day of pleasurable practice.

4. Forming Powerful, Transformative, Healing Images — Intentional mental imagery through Selective Awareness — Software For The Mind — allows you to make a commitment to healing yourself by directly influencing the behaviours of the cells of your body (e.g., the immune system), initiating and sustaining health-producing behaviours, (exercise, diet, non-abuse of alcohol or drugs, quit smoking), and produce a health-sustaining self-image. This inner image serves to change the behaviour at every level of the mind-body system.

5. Rehearsing These Images Daily — Reprogramming your mind is actually retraining the mind. Just as you might practice musical scales or typing in order to improve, the regular practice of the appropriate imagery trains the brain, the nervous system, and the immune system to easily carry out the desired changes. Your goal is to restore internal coherence and balance and thus to help heal the body, emotions, mind, and behavior.

6. Reinforcing Positive Changes — Reward your mind for responding to your entreaties so that the new behaviors prevail. Take yourself out for dinner, to a ball game, or a movie, for instance. Or take time off to be with loved ones.

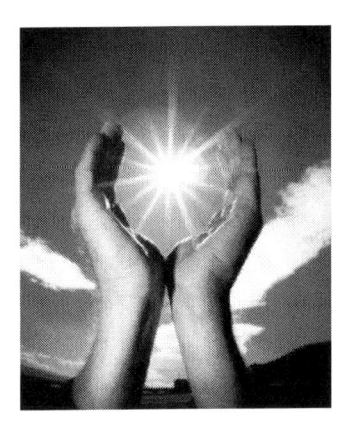

12. Mental Imagery and Role Models

By Gregg Swanson

The intention of this virtual personal coaching session is for you to write and answer these questions in your success journal and then reflect on them to gain insight on yourself, your dreams and what's holding you back.

Living a life of power, purpose and passion...with perseverance is walking the path of the Awakened Warrior. This path encompasses physical, emotional, spiritual and mental. The mental requires a mental strength mindset of empowering beliefs that will instil the feeling of empowerment.

Reaching your personal goals, achieving personal success and exceeding your human potential starts in your mind...and finishes with taking inspired and massive action.

12.1 Objective of this Mental Strength Tip:

To help you understand the power roles model can have in facilitating your way to reaching your personal goals and achieving personal success.

12.2 Modelling

An important key foundation in Neuro-linguistic Programming is modelling. To model, you emulate those who have already achieved success. You observe, analyze and then replicate the factors that contributed to the outstanding performance.

While there is no 100% guarantee that you can reap the same results, modelling helps you shorten your learning curve. You learn to avoid common mistakes and apply the essential steps and strategies that have helped your role model succeed. The idea is that it is much easier to follow a previously proven path to success.

12.3 Uncover Beliefs about Mental Thinking:

- In what areas of your life have you utilized roles models?
- Do you believe role models can expedite your personal success?
- If using roles models is so effective, why don't more people use them?

12.4 Unsupportive Beliefs about Role Models

- Role models are for children to admire.
- Role models are unapproachable.
- Role models are overrated.

12.5 Mental Strength Beliefs about Role Models

- Role models clear the path to success.
- Role models are fantastic teachers.
- Role models take the guesswork out of success.

12.6 Outrageous Questions:

- Who are your role models?
- Do you have role models in every area of your life?
- How many role models helped you get where you are today?

12.7 Reflective Questions:

- What would you have to do to find more role models for your life?
- How can I help you decided on new role models?
- How much time could you save by following the appropriate role models to manifest your life's purpose?

12.8 Mental Strength Coaching:

Role models are everywhere. Some are worthy of the term, others are thrust into the role for whatever reason and are not worthy of emulation by any stretch of the imagination. Yet it is human nature for all of us to seek out role models. We all want to see ourselves reflected in the faces of others who are successful and "just like us".

When you look for a role model, remember, they don't have to be "perfect" in every area of their life, only the area you want to emulate.

12.9 Final Thought

Any person, regardless of social stature, race, creed, and geographical location has looked up to someone for inspiration and aspire to be like him or her. People that motivate other people to do great things are role models. But role models need not come from the best schools, or have waged and won many wars, or have written tons of tomes that contemplate on man's existence; any person can be a role model to someone.

A role model serves as an inspiration or, as the case may be, a living guide to those who are inspired by his works, values, character, and life as a whole. Role models are pivotal to a person's success. College students, according to a study, were heavily influenced by their role models when deciding which career path they would likely take.

The criteria a person uses to choose a role model vary. Criteria are irrelevant in the grand scheme of things in one's life though, if a role model inspires one to do great things.

12.10 Role models are important.

They help us become the person we want to be and inspire us to make a difference. Choosing wisely means that you are influenced correctly and will help you be the best person you can be. To be like someone. you have to work hard.

Look for someone who is living life the way you would like to. If you want to be a famous author, your role model could be someone who has been successful at writing. If you have always wanted to be a nurse, your role model could be someone at your local hospital who is dedicated to their job and someone who you look up to for their achievements.

Look for key characteristics that you want to achieve. Choose a role model who may have done something you find admirable, such as raised a lot of money for charity, saved lots of lives, helped people in need or discovered the cure for a disease. Find someone who has good characteristics that you don't have (yet!). Here are some things to think about:

Choose someone who has a sense of purpose. A good role model would be someone who knows who they are. You don't want someone who seems perfect but doesn't have a sense of purpose. You want someone who won't pretend to be someone they are not and will not fake just to suit other people.

Consider someone who thinks it is all right to be unique, even if that means accepting some ridicule. They should make you feel good about being yourself, they shouldn't make you compare yourself to them and wish you were pretty.

Consider someone who interacts well with others, and someone who is kind and can communicate well with people. Like a teacher. People are easy to understand and emulate when they communicate well.

Consider someone who doesn't always take credit for what they do.

12.11 Focus on what is good..

Focus on what is good; don't emulate what is bad. Emulate him or her until you are a role model yourself; that's how you can know you have mastered the trait.

Keep in mind that having a role model does not mean you become exactly like that person. Remember to retain your individuality. Emulate them, but put your own individuality into the things they do.

True role models are those who possess the qualities that we would like to have. Role models are also those who have affected us in a way that makes us want to be better people. Sometimes, we don't recognize people we are emulating until we have noticed our own personal growth and progress that they have caused.

Still listen to other people. Sometimes we can be blind to our own mistakes, and we can emulate bad characteristics. Accept others' ideas well so that you don't make the same mistakes that they might have made.

Some poorly chosen role models may take advantage of their position and make you do things to make you look bad or a very bad influence to others. Make sure that you don't follow one and emulate someone without thought.

Make sure to remember that people are imperfect.

12.12 How To Choose The Right Role Model

This will probably disappoint you: there is no such thing as a perfect role model.

Nobody is perfect. Being perfect means to be done with this world, even literally if you look at the word 'perfect' and its etymology.

So, all we can hope for is that we choose at least a 'good' role model.

A 'good' role model is one that makes it easy for you to adopt. We'll learn about three common mistakes one can make while working with his or her role model later in this article.

So, where can one find a role model? This is easy since we've got marvellous technology at our disposal. We can utilize magazines, newspapers, books, movies, cds, dvds, our tv and of course the internet.

But if you want to become more effective you first have to figure out how exactly you want to be. It's wise to write down how you want to be after the role model process. By writing it down you can analyze your progress later and adjust the number and kind of your role models.

This sounds all a bit technical, I know. But becoming more effective is not some kind of magic. Everybody can become more effective with this simple method. It sounds technical because it IS technical. It's a skill, a craft you have to learn in order to utilize it.

So, in order to choose the right role model you have to choose people who are good at what they're doing. You have to choose people who inspire you.

If you want to be a famous singer you have to choose a famous singer as your role model. If you want to become more successful at work you have to choose a successful co-worker whom you admire for his abilities. If you want to be a better parent you have to look for parents that you ask for advice when you need it. If you want to be beautiful you have to find people who are beautiful.

Finding the right role model is pretty easy. The next part is harder.

Giordano Bruno

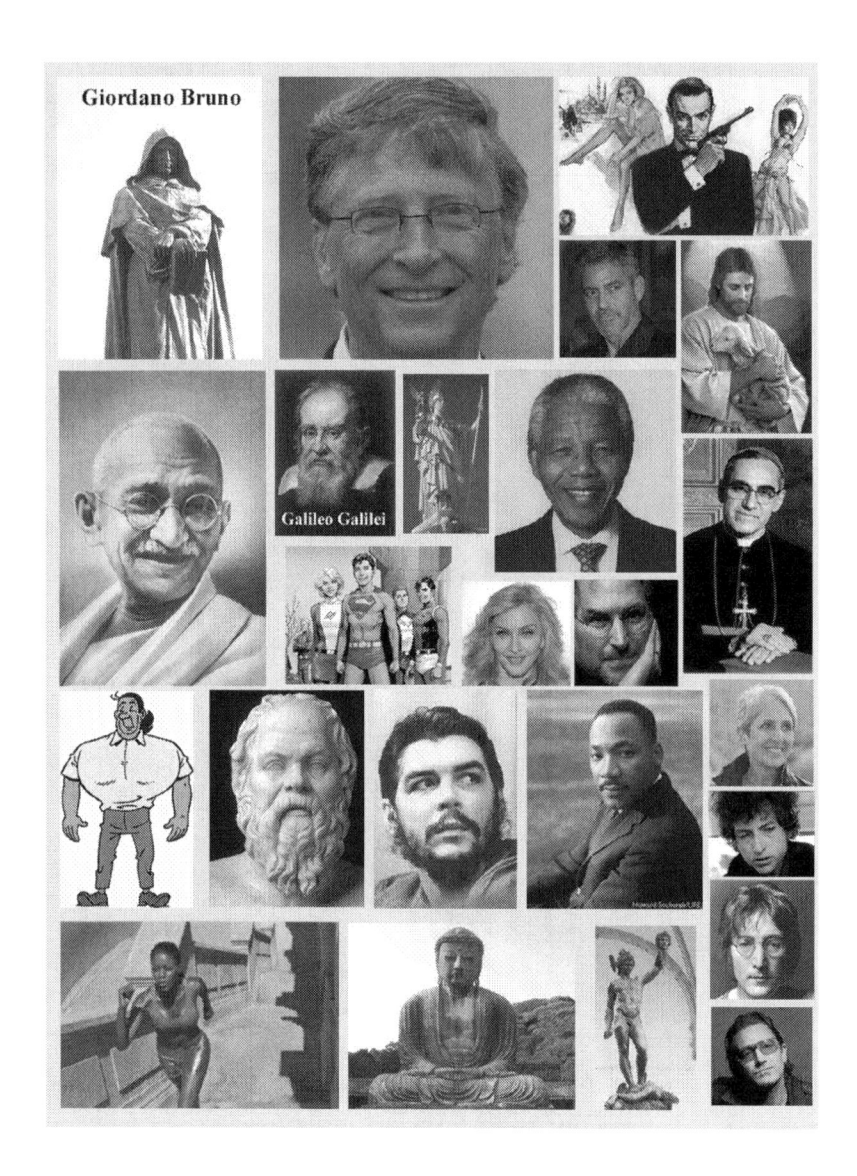

Galileo Galilei

12.13 How To Become Who You Want To Be

I suppose you get the idea of choosing a role model for your purposes. Now you want to become more effective, finally. How do you do it? This will sound easy, but it isn't: in order to become who you want to be you have to alter your point of view first.

You have to detach yourself from yourself. Well, that sounds weird, doesn't it? What I mean is this: while you're making progress you'll encounter a lot of problems which might make you want to stop the whole thing and return to your 'normal' life.

You are who you are and changing this is impossible. Our ego 'thinks' we are better off with our 'old self' so it's interfering whenever it can.

Let's assume that you want to become more effective at your job, thus more successful. In order to do so you have to adopt the skills that your role model utilizes to be successful. This might include working late. But working late is a no-no for you. So, now you're screwed because instead of encouraging you to keep the pace and overcome your 'I-don't-want-to-work-late-issues' your ego will say something like this: "If THIS is what it takes, I'll quit."

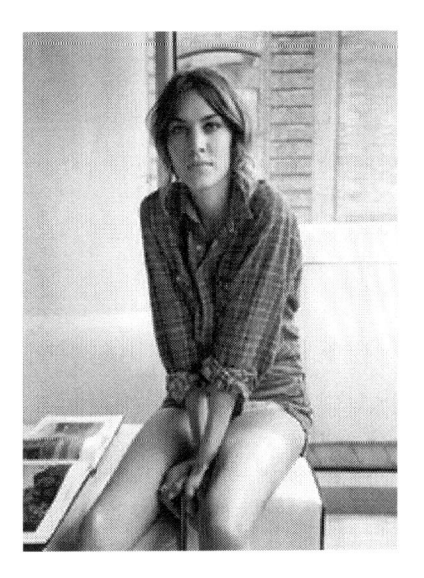

Don't give in though. This is totally normal, you just have to remember how the outcome will feel like. You'll have to motivate yourself. A lot.

12.14 Examples.

Example 1: Being beautiful

Being beautiful is one of the strongest desires among millions on our planet Earth. In order to be more effective regarding beauty you now have to adopt the set of abilities that certain beautiful people have.

This means you have to answer the following questions:
- which beauty products do they use?
- what and how much do they eat?
- what's their recipe for happiness?
- which 'soft skills' have they learned?

The above list of questions or better yet: quests is not complete. You have to find out what makes these people beautiful. And you have to answer yourself why you (!) perceive them as beautiful since this is totally subjective and only meaningful for you alone.

Example 2: Being successful

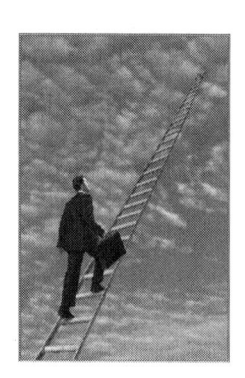

Being successful probably means something different for you than it does for me. It may translate into having a lot of money, leading a huge company, driving fast cars, eating out every day, wearing delicate clothes but it could also mean to write a book, create a wonderful garden or to bring peace to the world.

You have to choose role models that you consider to be successful and you'll have to answer questions like these:

- do they have a MBA?
- who were their mentors?
- when do they get up in the morning?
- how did they get their ideas?

And again the list of questions is not complete. Find out as much as possible about your role model in order to adopt as many skills as possible.

Example 3: Being healthy

Being healthy is also a very popular 'dream' of millions. Most of us don't think about it consciously because we have things like health insurances and cities crowded with doctors of all kinds. If you're sick you have to find role models who are extremely healthy.

If you answer the following (and a lot more) questions it will be easier for you to understand why these people are healthy:

- do they smoke, drink or eat junk food?
- which books did they read in order to get healthy?
- how do they manage to stay healthy (not only physically)?
- have they been in touch with some kind of faith healer?

As you can see human desires are wide-spread. We all want different things. But in order to get what we want we all have to follow the rules. You can become more effective by choosing the right role model.

You have to think of a way to overcome yourself and move on. Do it now.

12.15 Four Common Mistakes

I've already mentioned that you might stumble upon a few problems during the metamorphosis. That's quite normal and most issues will vanish on its own. But four of these mistakes can be pretty grave so

I'll explain how you can avoid them or at least deal with them when it's already 'too late'.

Mistake #1 – You try to become your role model

You cannot become another human being. At least not physically. If you try to become your role model you are bound to fail. You can only adopt the abilities and the mindset of your role model.

You want to be a famous actor? Fine. You can do it. But you cannot become Christian Bale. He's already there. You can become somebody who has a similar mindset and similar abilities but you can never be him.

Mistake #2 – You force yourself to become somebody you can't connect with

Sometimes we dream about an alternate version of our lives and forget about the big picture. Let's say you picked an actor as your role model and you find out that he's been doing pornographic movies in his early years. You do not have to copy this if you don't like it. It's about the abilities and the mindset of your role model, it's not really about their specific (and personal) actions.

Mistake #3 – You adopt a 'bad lifestyle'

In the beginning of this article I told you about a 'good' role model and now I'm talking about a 'bad' lifestyle – whether you perceive something as good or bad is your business and your business alone.

But when you begin to feel bad during your metamorphosis it's very likely that you've lost your track. It's important to get back on track otherwise the whole process would be pointless.

Just because your role model smokes 20 cigarettes per day that does not mean that you have to adopt this behaviour as well. The secret to a clean metamorphosis is that you make conscious decisions about what you want to adopt from your role model and what not.

Smoking is not healthy and if you want to stay healthy but also want to be successful as an actor you can just ignore the role model's frailties. Pick what will make you happy. Ignore the rest.

Mistake #4 – You give up too early

This whole process can take weeks, months, even years so you should brace yourself for this adventure. Don't give up just because you don't get quick results. You want permanent results, don't you? You want to be and STAY successful, you want to be and STAY beautiful, you want to be and STAY healthy.

Don't get blinded by temporary results. Look at your notes from the beginning. What exactly was your goal? Adjust your plan if needed.

Your Personal Strengths & Role Models

Based on the premise that what you notice and greatly appreciate in others is also within you, we invite you to bring to the fore your role models.

List 3 qualities or strengths for each of your Top 5 role models. Choose anyone who has lived or is currently living. You may even nominate a fictional childhood hero.

Draw a table or grid with two columns, one for the names of the role models and the other for their respective strengths.

Once completed, scan the strengths and notice any repetition or distinctive ones.

For example, does DECISIVE appear three times? Is INSPIRING a quality that you really admire even though it shows up only once?

There is a chance that both are strengths of yours although they may need a hint of honing.

Make a shortlist of those strengths that speak to you loudly and that you feel would be particularly rewarding if they were leveraged more regularly, meaningfully, or intentionally.

Be attentive to what resonates with you most.

Commit to taking two actions/strength over the next week that will create value in your life.

Insert them in your agenda to ensure follow through.

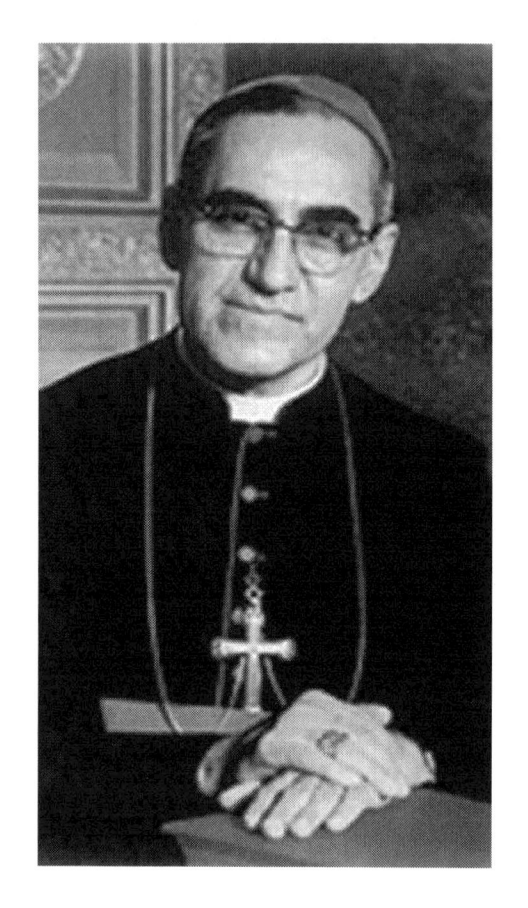

Source:

http://www.warriormindcoach.com/blog/2013/04/01/mental-strength-tip-133-role-models-for-personal-success/

13. How to Think Like a Genius

Edited by KnowItSome, Bo, LB.StorM, Chris Hadley and 56 others

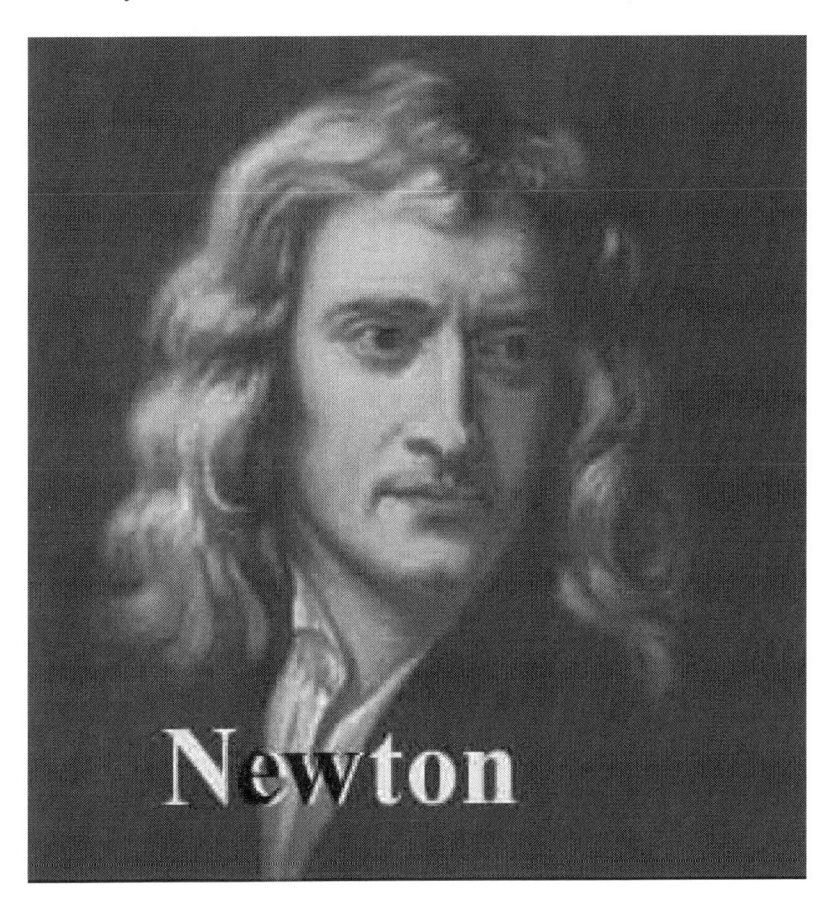

There are many ways to classify a genius. But if you look at the historical figures whom most people would consider geniuses, such as Albert Einstein, Leonardo Da Vinci, and Beethoven, you can see one thing they all share in common: they were all able to think in a way different from the mainstream, and thus made connections that no one else did. Based on that pattern, this article will address some of the ways you can think like a genius.

13.1 Steps

1 Love learning.

Geniuses are passionate about the things they do. If you want to think like a genius, find what you love and dive in headfirst.

Figure out what your learning style is and make use of it. The major types are auditory, visual-spatial, verbal-linguistic and kinaesthetic. Experiment with different techniques for absorbing information and stick with what works best.

Learn how to self-educate. There are lots of resources available on the internet and through local services like community colleges and libraries that can put all sorts of exciting information at your fingertips.

Be pro-active and ask questions. There are people you meet every day that know all sorts of things and have all sorts of valuable skills to share. As a genius, be interested in the potential in everything.

Be over-comprehensive in your studies. Learn everything there is to know.

As you learn about different disciplines, think about how they connect to one another.

2. Start ambitious projects and see them through from start to finish.

Genius ideas have often occurred in the pursuit of something that many contemporaries thought to be downright crazy. Create opportunities for yourself to discover new things by embarking on journeys no one has embarked on yet.

3. Embrace change, uncertainty, and doubt.

It is on these edges of knowledge that innovation and discovery happen. Don't be afraid to question conventional wisdom; geniuses are the ones who rewrite those conventions.

4. Be prolific.

Try for quantity before quality. To produce exceptionally good work, do a lot of whatever you're doing. It increases your chances for success and it means you will get more practice along the way. It also takes the pressure off, knowing that while an effort may be your first, it will likely not be your last. Most geniuses in history, whatever they were doing, did a LOT of it, and not all of it was genius!

There is a theory that to become a "master" in any subject, you need 10,000 hours of practice. Professional orchestra players, computer programmers all demonstrate this idea. (Citation: Malcolm Gladwell's book Outliers, 2009, but see also Creativity: Genius and other Myths, Weisberg, 1986)

5. Learn about Bloom's Taxonomy.

Bloom's Taxonomy is a breakdown of the six levels of thinking, from the lowest level to the highest. You can use it to help you think about thinking on a deeper level.

Knowledge is accepting and believing a fact. Knowing $2 + 2 = 4$, doesn't mean you know what $2 + 2 = 4$ means.

Application is knowing how to use the fact. You can determine that 2 cats plus 2 cats equals 4 cats. You don't know what $2 + 2 = 4$ means, but you can apply it.

Comprehension is understanding a fact: You understand the concept of addition and how $2 + 2 = 4$.

Analysis is breaking down information into its parts. 4 - 2 = 2 ; (1 + 1) + (1 + 1) = 2 + 2 = 4

Synthesis is Creating something new. (2 + 2) + (2 + 2) = 4 + 4

Evaluation: Discussion of the merits of 2 + 2 = 4.

6. Think differently.

You are different. You think differently. Every kind of genius IS different and individual. And every kind of opinion has something true and something you can learn from.

Remember that different ideas have not historically been accepted well, and yours may not be either. Geniuses throughout history have not let this deter them; neither should you.

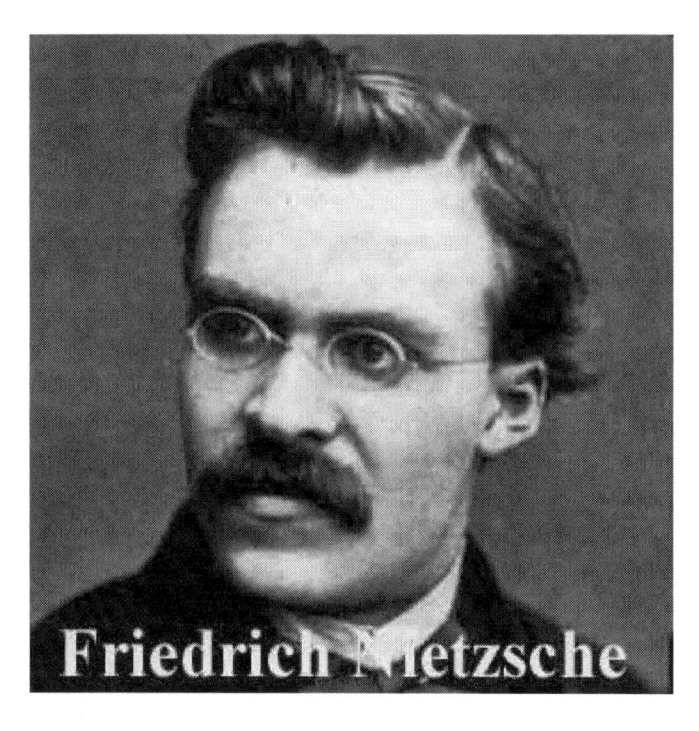

Friedrich Nietzsche

Choose an image and it relate it to your life.
1. Give an example of a connection you have made to the image.
2. Think about what the image tells you about work and life.
3. Create a plan that will make a change.
4. Apply this change to your work and life.

Tips

- Learn to take suggestions and criticisms in a positive way. Many things can be learned from intelligent people if you listen to them.
- Read about geniuses, especially in the field(s) that interest you. What made Richard Feynman great? What about Thomas Edison?
- If you think you are almost as smart as a genius set even higher goal for yourself.
- Do not read only about geniuses, but also read what geniuses wrote, so that you can see how they were thinking. Always search for primary sources.

Source

http://www.wikihow.com/Think-Like-a-Genius

Metaphorming: The Official "Think Like a Genius"® Method[1]

This is an outline of a method that is taught in workshops and discussed in the book "Think Like a Genius" by Dr. Todd Siler. It involves connecting and transforming information (data, knowledge, concepts, experiences, etc.) in personally meaningful, purposeful and useful ways.

14. Visualisation Boards

14.1 Personality Boards

At some point in our lives, the question will arise: Who am I NOW?

A personality board is an ideal tool to remind us of the different aspects of our personality as they result from introspection and from various personality tests.

Unless we use the board only for looking back at how we felt ourselves during a particular moment in our lives, it is important to choose for a formulae that allows for easy adaption. Some parts of our personality will normally remain unchanged during all or most of our lives as a result of conscious or subconscious changes and adaptations such as may be triggered by changes in our environment.

In fact we are all more or less influenced by personal and social experiences as friends, partners, profession, age, health, life-style, personal successes and failures all leave their mark on us. A personality board is very helpful to easily remind us of the preferences and choices we expressed at a given time in our lives

Steps

1. Create a neutral background either on computer or on an actual board.

2. Select images that reflect personality and character traits you identify yourself with. Pay special attention to elements that feel familiar or make you feel emotional.

3. Print your personality board and hang it to the wall at a place where it will be in sight or use it as a computer desktop wallpaper.

Tamara's Personality Board at age 16

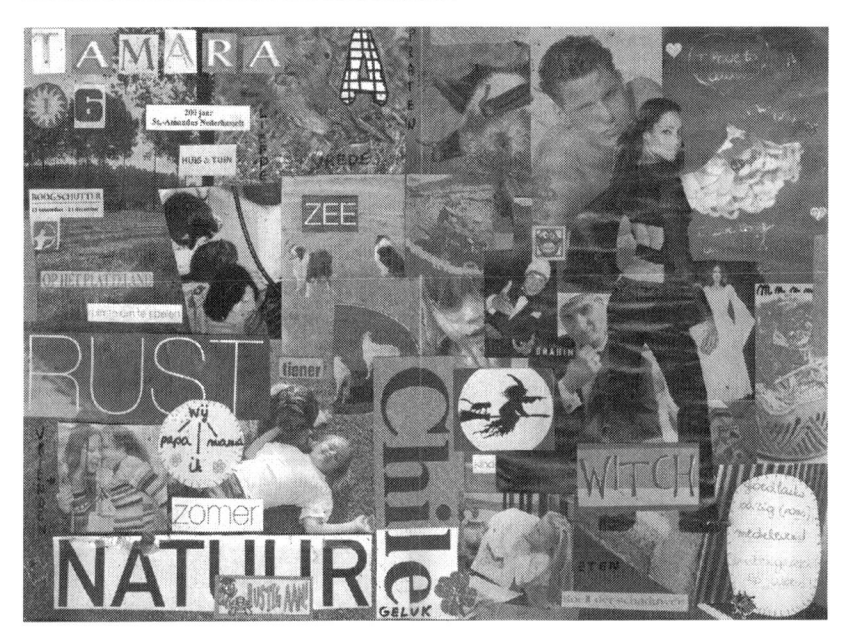

Eddy's Personality Board

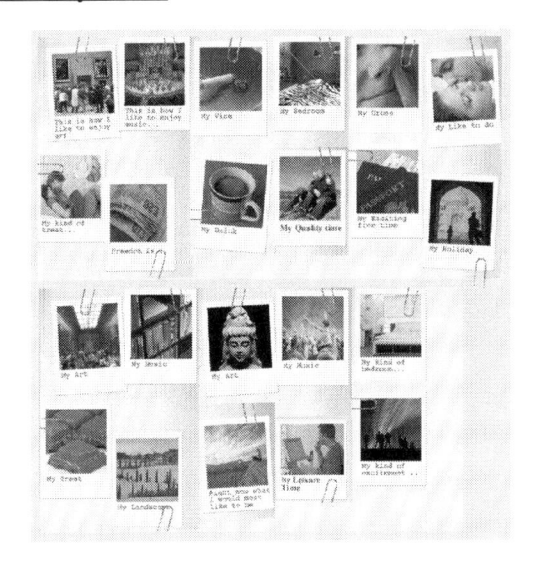

Tips:

Feel free to select images from any field that is important to you.

Some possibilities are: lifestyle, sports, fitness and wellness, clothes, make-up, meals, drinks, houses, restaurants, cars, preferred leisure time, vacation, city trips, profession, hobbies, role-models, cartoons, politicians, spiritual preferences, pets, animal totems, achievements, strong points, challenges, likes, MBTI-personality type, Enneagram type, favourite quotes, art, movies, music, desired future, precious memories ...

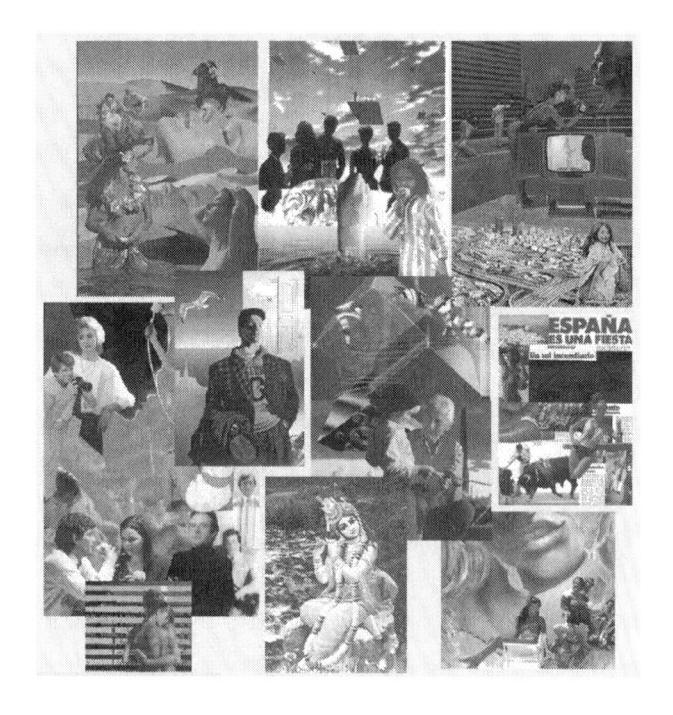

Important is that, when you look at your personality board, you find yourself reflected in the images you selected. Images which, of course, you are free to replace by others at any time you feel that they do not longer correctly reflect who you are and how you think and feel.

14.2 Vision Boards or Dream Boards

A vision board is a collage of images, pictures and affirmations of your dreams and desires. It can also be called a dream board, treasure map or vision map.

Vision boards are a great way to make you feel positive, and are helpful if you are using the law of attraction.

Steps:

1. Decide the main theme of your board. It may be based on something specific you wish to accomplish or obtain, or it may be a general idea of everything that makes you happy and that you want to see in your future.
2. Find pictures that correspond with your theme
3. Print (if necessary) and cut out your pictures, then glue them to your vision board or arrange them on your computer-made board.
4. Type or write some affirmations that correspond with your theme.
5. Hang your vision board in a place you will see every day or use it as your computer desktop wallpaper.
6. View your board at least once a day, and focus on the objects, sayings and theme of your board.

Tips

Don't be afraid to change your board to reflect more specific thoughts, or a new theme.

You may wish to place a picture of yourself in the centre as it shows you being surrounded by the things you desire.

Only attach pictures that pertain to your theme. You should even pay attention to small unwanted items in the background of pictures.

14.3 The Power of Vision Boards

BY JESSICA SEPEL

A vision board is a simple yet powerful visualization tool that manifests your dreams into reality by activating the Law of Attraction.

Oprah Winfrey and many other highly successful people have used this technique for generations. It consists of a poster or foam board of cut-out pictures, drawings and phrases of the things that you want in your life, or the things that you want to become.

Some examples include: pictures of places you would like to travel, your favourite car, dream lover, your dream body, your business goals, inspirational quotes, pictures of friends and family... really anything that you love and you are grateful for.

The idea behind this is that when you surround yourself with positive images of who you want to become, what you want to have, where you want to live and the things you are grateful for, your life changes to match those images and those desires. The law of attraction in essence! When we express gratitude, we bring more into our lives to be thankful for. Although it may seem otherwise at times, we all have many things to be grateful for. If you are reading this blog, then you can be grateful for your eyesight and for being able to read!

I made a vision board about two years ago. I placed phrases and pictures of things I wanted to achieve onto it. I kept it on my desk; so every day when I walked through my room I would glance at my goals and dreams. Now looking at it two years later, I can truly tell you that 80 or 90 percent of the things I placed on the board have become my reality. And a very happy reality, too!

The Power of Vision Boards
BY JANE MORRIS

Vision boards have transformed the lives of celebrities like Arnold Schwarzenegger and Oprah Winfrey – and they have the power to transform your life too. They are a modern manifestation method combining concepts taken from creative hobbies like scrapbooking with motivational mind-mapping and brand development techniques used by marketers. A vision board is quite literally a collage of pictures, phrases, poems and quotes visually represent what you would like to experience more of in your life. An increasing number of Hollywood celebrities, Olympic athletes, television personalities and top motivational speakers have started to share how vision boards help sustain their success. Vision Boards are fast being recognised as more than just a bit of creative fun, and credited by leaders of our time a powerful tool for transformation. From Barack Obama's Campaign Manager to Olympian Rueben Gonzalez vision boards are helping millions of people worldwide to manifest their dreams.

But vision boards don't work for everyone. This is because most people make the mistake of beginning a board without first connecting to their inner wisdom. The result is a board filled with images and words that aren't aligned to their authentic desires. If a vision board only contains pictures of what the ego thinks it wants then it won't be effective. For a vision board to attract like a magnet it is important for it to be created with gratitude, positive intention, self-acceptance and a sense of flow. In order to begin the process relax your body, and mind and turn your attention within.

If you find yourself predominantly being drawn towards images of items you'd like to own, then it's probably your ego creating a shopping list, rather than your soul expressing its fullest vision for yourself. A simple way to escape your ego is to ask yourself "what more would I want?" every time you run into something that feels like it comes from outside of yourself or represents someone else's dream goal for you. Each time you ask yourself this question you'll get closer and closer to the higher vision your heart holds for you.

The pictures you stick on your board may come from things in your outside environment like magazines and brochures, but you need your inner navigation system to guide you intuitively to the images and phrases that will inspire you and ignite the power of your board. Let the feeling of happiness in your heart help you find pictures that mirror what you'd most like to manifest in your life.

Another common vision board blunder is to create a collage crammed with 'wishful thinking' rather than overflowing with belief that you can truly have whatever you put on your board. Before any images are selected and stuck down it is important to have cleared out any limiting beliefs that may stop you from believing you have the power to enjoy the presence of your desired experience, person, place or thing in your life. If you don't believe that you are entitled to or can bring about the things you placed on your board, then you will block them from coming to you. But if you release any negative thoughts and emotion, and create your board feeling inspired, excited and enthused, then your board will be super-charged with the positive energy of your true potential.

Once completed it is crucial to hang your board somewhere that you actively spend the majority of your day. Poor positioning is something can completely stifle vision board success. Many people create beautiful boards filled with inspiring images that celebrate their greatest vision for themselves, then hide the board in a cupboard or hang it up in a room they never use. For your board to truly bring abundant blessings it needs to be located at eye level in a space where it can be admired and appreciated regularly. The best place to hang your board is in your office or living room. The more time you spend with your board the more movement you will make toward your goals and the faster they will manifest into reality.

If you'd like to start the new year with a new vision for a new you, then a vision board is a powerful way to take stock on where you are at in your life and reflect on what you would like to do differently during the year ahead. Follow these 7 Simple Steps and discover how to take time for yourself, let go of all the things that didn't work out in the past, acknowledge the powerful creator within you, align your vision with the life you'd love to live and support yourself in stepping forward with confidence and clarity into 2011.

Tips:

Mindset Magic – Let go of anything you feel you 'should, ought to or must' aspire towards. Give yourself permission to explore the things that you really want to welcome more of in your life.

You don't need to know what the images represent for you at this stage. Simply focus on keeping all the images you love looking at and trust your intuition on any pictures that don't feel right. Sift through the pile so that only the images and words that really inspire you remain.

Ask yourself : "What would I like to be, do or have in my life if I knew it was okay to have anything I wanted? If I knew I deserved it? If I had full support from others? If I knew I could succeed? If I had no fear? If I had abundant resources and all the time I needed?"

Mission Statement – Connect with your sense of purpose and write a mission statement to summarise what it is you want to manifest in your life. If you are uncertain of what your mission in life is, take yourself back to your memories of how you enjoyed spending time as a child. Often we expressed the essence of our life purpose in the things that intrigued and occupied us as children. Also in the dreams we had of what we wanted to do when we 'grew up'.

Take three deep breaths, turn your focus inward and ask yourself "what am I here to do". Notice what thoughts, feelings or sensations you get. Write your mission statement in the first person, e.g. "I am an inspirational teacher, making a positive difference in the lives of underprivileged children". Underneath your mission statement write the things you will experience as you actualize this vision of yourself, e.g. "I am happy and healthy. I have wonderful relationships. I experience abundance in all areas of my life. I enjoy giving and receiving love".

Write your mission statement accompanied by a current photo of yourself at the centre of your board.

Then experiment by arranging all your other images on your board in whatever way feels good. Move them around until you are happy, then stick or fix them in place. There is no right or wrong way to secure your images. Trust your gut feeling. The important thing is to arrange your images with plenty of space in between, so that you send out a message to the universe that you are always open to receiving more!

Position with Pride – Proudly display your board somewhere in your home or office where you are most active during the day and will see it regularly (even if this is from your peripheral vision). Position it at eye level in a space that is in alignment with your vision – i.e. not above your toilet or inside a cupboard! Ensure the space around your board supports your vision, clear away any clutter or things that don't reflect the words and images on your board.

Ongoing Process – Allow your vision board to be a continuously moving creation with room to add more images as your ideas develop and change. Whenever you bring something on your board into being celebrate and express gratitude for this success :) pop a little smiley face next to the word or image, make a tick mark or write 'thank you!'.

Sources:

http://www.wikihow.com/Make-a-Vision-Board

http://www.mindbodygreen.com/0-5824/The-Power-of-Vision-Boards.html

http://www.selfgrowth.com/articles/the-power-of-vision-boards

Jayne Morris, The POWER Coach, is Founder and Director of Power-Up™, the unique coaching system combining life coaching, meditation, visualization, martial arts, angelic healing and integrative art therapy. Jayne is an expert in helping busy, successful women do less and be more. Jayne helps her clients connect with their inner power, passions and potential, enabling them to pursue their dreams and make positive change. To get your FREE Power-Up Energiser Meditation and receive her eZine featuring high quality self development articles visit www.jaynemorris.com

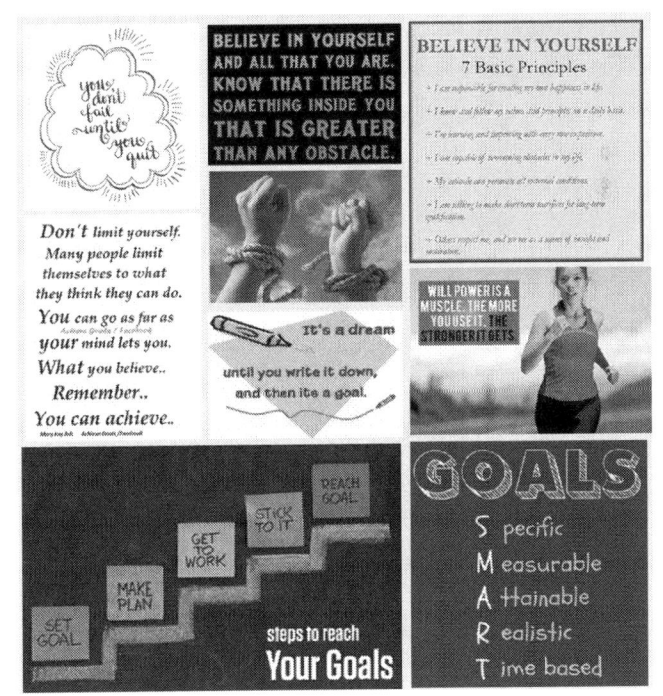

14.4 Action Boards

BY REPORTING TJ

Every now and then, often around New Year, you may find yourself thinking about your resolutions. With time, however, some of us quit making them because we never stick to them. That's me. I make them but then quickly forget what they were or lose focus. Vision boards have been around forever but recently the "trend" emerged to replace them by "Action Boards".

Why the change? Well: Vision boards are based on the Law of Attraction. The idea that your mode of thinking directly affects what the universe gives you. So, cutting out pictures and writing down positive affirmations can be beneficial and can help organize your goals. But if your board is filled with fantasy, it can set you up for failure. Some psychologists say instead of making a "Vision Board" make an "Action Board". If you ask me I think they are basically the same thing. I mean, let's be realistic just imagining you are going to get that new bedroom set you've REALLY wanted isn't going to just poof magically appear in your bedroom. You have to actually save the money for said bedroom set. So, if I look at the bedroom set every day it's a top of mind reminder that I don't need Starbucks, I can make my own coffee and put that $5.00 away to save for that bedroom set. Makes Sense?

To make an action board you select images of things you want to change, get or do, and paste them to the board. Next, you hang the board somewhere you can see it all the time every day to keep your goals top of mind.

Remember just having arts and crafts day at your house won't help make your dreams come true but it can help you visualize them. Don't make it super cluttered, I've seen vision boards with ALL kinds of things on there. How can you focus on one goal at a time with all that clutter?! You can't. So post 4 or 5 pictures of things and goals that are actually attainable.

You aren't going to marry Channing Tatum in 2013, sorry. Don't cut out pictures of Obama if you want to be president. You aren't going to Freaky Friday switch places with him in 2013. Be simple. Maybe instead of cutting out a picture of Channing Tatum, you write "go on dates with dark haired guys who can dance" or if you do want to be president write "delete facebook, ask friends to erase/give back incriminating photos" think baby steps. simple. attainable.

My point is... No matter what you call it, a picture board only works if you take action to complete those goals and if you are like me and forget your resolutions or give up after a month or two, maybe making one of these is something you could try!

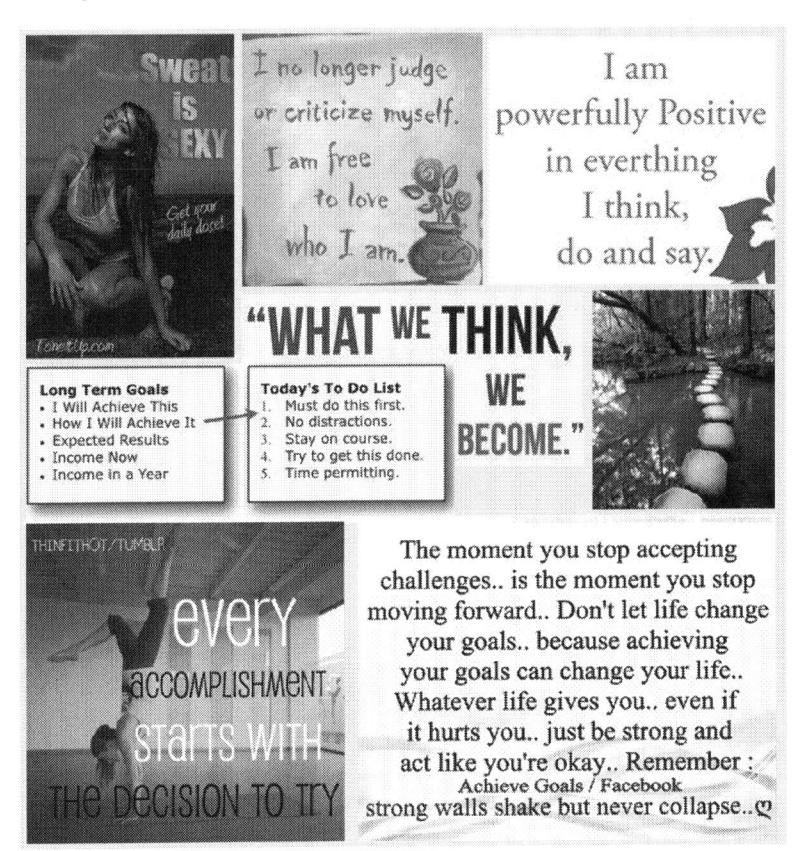

Sweat is Sexy
Get your daily dose!

I no longer judge or criticize myself. I am free to love who I am.

I am powerfully Positive in everthing I think, do and say.

"WHAT WE THINK, WE BECOME."

Long Term Goals
- I Will Achieve This
- How I Will Achieve It
- Expected Results
- Income Now
- Income in a Year

Today's To Do List
1. Must do this first.
2. No distractions.
3. Stay on course.
4. Try to get this done.
5. Time permitting.

every accomplishment starts with the decision to try

The moment you stop accepting challenges.. is the moment you stop moving forward.. Don't let life change your goals.. because achieving your goals can change your life.. Whatever life gives you.. even if it hurts you.. just be strong and act like you're okay.. Remember :
Achieve Goals / Facebook
strong walls shake but never collapse..

14.5 Throw Away Your Vision Board

BY NEIL FARBER,

Published in The Blame Game

Vision boards are for dreaming, action boards are for achieving.

Vision or Dream boards have achieved notoriety in the past few years with the release of the book, The Secret. An endorsement from Oprah also didn't hurt. Vision boards are based on the Law of Attraction. The idea that your mode of thinking directly affects what the universe gives you. If you put positive mental energy into the universe, you'll be the recipient of positive outcomes.

The Law of Attraction is not new. Before The Secret, there was the book, Creative Visualization which described the same phenomenon. As classically taught, the Law of Attraction is universal and as such, always works if you do it correctly. Thus, the reason for any unrealized goals is that you did not provide enough positive thoughts and energy to the process or you let some negative thoughts slip in. In short, you're completely to blame for your lack of success.

Creating your own vision board is considered the key to success. It is not enough to simply have a positive mental attitude. The secret to achieving your goals is to dream about positive, focused, and specific goals.

As The Complete Idiot's Guide to Vision Boards describes, the images and phrases that make the board should represent your highest priorities. Some posit that a certain amount of time spent in front of the board is necessary for complete success, while others suggest that simply creating the vision board is what is critical to maintain the goal in your subconscious. If you think about your goals as if they've already occurred, then the universe will give this to you.

Here's my take on Vision Boards.

Cutting out pictures and writing down positive affirmations may be beneficial to some; in particular, helping us organize and more clearly delineate our goals. However, there is good evidence that these actions may also be detrimental.

The evidence:

Experiment #1.

(from Pham and Taylor at the Univ of Ca):

Three groups of students: Group 1 (Secret group – my label not from the study): students were asked to spend a few moments each day visualizing with a clear image how great it would feel to make a high grade on an important mid-term exam that would take place in a few days time. Group 2: students were asked to spend a few minutes each day visualizing when, where, and how they intended to study. Group 3: control group of students not asked to visualize doing especially well on the exams. Students visualizing being A students (Group 1), studied less and made lower grades on the exam. They felt better about themselves but achieved less. Students visualizing studying, prepared better, studied more, scored higher grades, and were less stressed.

Experiment #2.

(Pham and Taylor).

A similar studied showed similar results for golfers and tennis players. They were more successful if they imagined themselves training rather than winning.

Experiment #3.

(from Oettingen and Wadden at the Univ Penn):

A group of obese women in a weight reduction program were asked to imagine how they might behave in various food-related scenarios, such as being tempted with pizza. Their responses were categorized on a scale from highly positive (e.g. I would stay away from cake and ice cream) to highly negative (e.g. I would be eating both my own and other people's portions). The women were tracked for a year. Those with more positive fantasies had lost, on average, 26 lbs less than those with negative fantasies.

Experiment #4.

(Oettingen):

A group of students with a serious crush on a classmate were asked to imagine what would happen in various scenarios, such as arriving early to class and seeing the door open and the object of their desire enter. The degree of their fantasizing was rated as positive (eg Our eyes meet and we both know that this is the type of love that happens once in a lifetime) to negative (we are both free and single, he turns to me, smiles and asks how I am. For reasons that I still do not fully understand, I explain that I already have a boyfriend.) Five months later, those with positive fantasies were less likely to have been forthcoming about their crush or made other overtures toward having a relationship with them.

Experiment #5.

(Oettingen).

Senior students were asked to note how often they fantasized about getting their dream job after college graduation. Two-year follow-up — the students who had frequently fantasized about success had submitted fewer job applications, received fewer job offers, and had smaller salaries.

Some thoughts:

1) Positive mental attitudes, dreaming, wishing, and fantasizing may, in fact, be harmful.

2) We are in control of our own thoughts, feelings, actions, and reactions. We have no control over the actions of others.

3) The universe may have other plans. We don't know if there are other, greater plans behind the curtain. Thus, not achieving our goals may actually be beneficial for us. The outcome, while apparently negative, may be a blessing in disguise. Rather than blaming yourself, you would be better off finding the silver lining, looking for lessons learned and realizing how this apparent failure can be beneficial.

4) Two people may have the same vision and only one person can achieve a goal – winning a race or owning a specific house. For the person not achieving the goal, rather than self-blame, time would be better spent looking for reasons for the lack of success, rearranging their dominoes to change course, and moving on to better things.

5) According to the Law of Attraction, if you think about and plan for potential obstacles, and your goal is not realized, you will be to blame for including negativity and doubt. If you don't look at and plan for potential obstacles, you will be unprepared mentally, emotionally, and practically for facing real challenges.

6) Ideas, thoughts, and dreams are great, but they are forms of energy which do not necessarily lead to action.

7) It's easier to think, wish, and dream than to do.

Action vs Dreaming

"Do it, and then you will feel motivated to do it." - Zig Ziglar

"Good business leaders create a vision, articulate the vision, passionately own the vision, and relentlessly drive it to completion." - Jack Welch

"The secret of getting ahead is getting started." - Mark Twain

"As I grow older I pay less attention to what men say. I just watch what they do." - Andrew Carnegie

"Everything you want is out there waiting for you to ask. Everything you want also wants you. But you have to take action to get it." - Jules Renau

"I never worry about action, but only about inaction." - Winston Churchill.

"I have been impressed with the urgency of doing. Knowing is not enough; we must apply. Being willing is not enough; we must do." – Leonardo da Vinci

"Vision without action is a dream. Action without vision is simply passing the time. Action with Vision is making a positive difference." - Joel Barker

Conclusion: Fantasizing about your perfect world and your perfect life may make you feel better in the short term but will limit your ability to transform your dreams into reality. Convert your vision boards to action boards.

Dream about it, envision how you will realistically do it or get it, and then get off your tusk and make it happen.

Visual + Action...Board

BY GRETCHEN FOGELSTROM

Next Saturday I am getting together with friends and we are planning on creating Vision Boards.

So in preparation, as I have not done this before, I thought it would be interesting to learn more about the psychology of this act and what others are saying out there.

This morning I have been doing a bit of research and it seems that ONLY visualizing, dreaming, and thinking positive thoughts may actually lull us into non-doing, sitting back and waiting...taking the easy road, all to find that we are still dreaming of what we want rather than achieving the outcome we envision.

Digging a bit deeper I also found that taking action without having a goal, the big dream, or a vision of what the result will be is also a detriment to getting what or where we want to be as we are not focused.

Over the last couple of weeks I have been slowly reading through "The Happiness Project" by Gretchen Rubin. I have found it very inspiring, even though my life and circumstances are quite different from her's. I too feel happy but want to be happier. In "The Happiness Project", she outlines how making specific, small tasks a regular habit is very important. From getting in at least 30 minutes a day with your heart-rate elevated to a 10 minute nightly "tidy" up of the house – whatever works for you of course, but the focus is on the small. Small things that make a big difference de-cluttering your mind and energizing your body... more happiness. I like this way of thinking as I can implement my list more easily. Having the big goal of losing 20lbs is, well, depressing. But getting my heart-rate up for 30 minutes a day is doable.

So visualizing the goal but with actionable steps to get there makes a lot of sense to me. So I think Saturday's vision board is now going to be a VISUAL~ACTION Board.

Have you ever created a Vision/Dream Board? Did you see results? Ever created an Action Board? I'd love to hear what you've created and how it worked for you.

I'll update you after our Saturday fun. Oh – and we're going Conga dancing after we finish our boards – so should be a fun night of talking about where we want to go with our lives and then shaking ourselves silly!

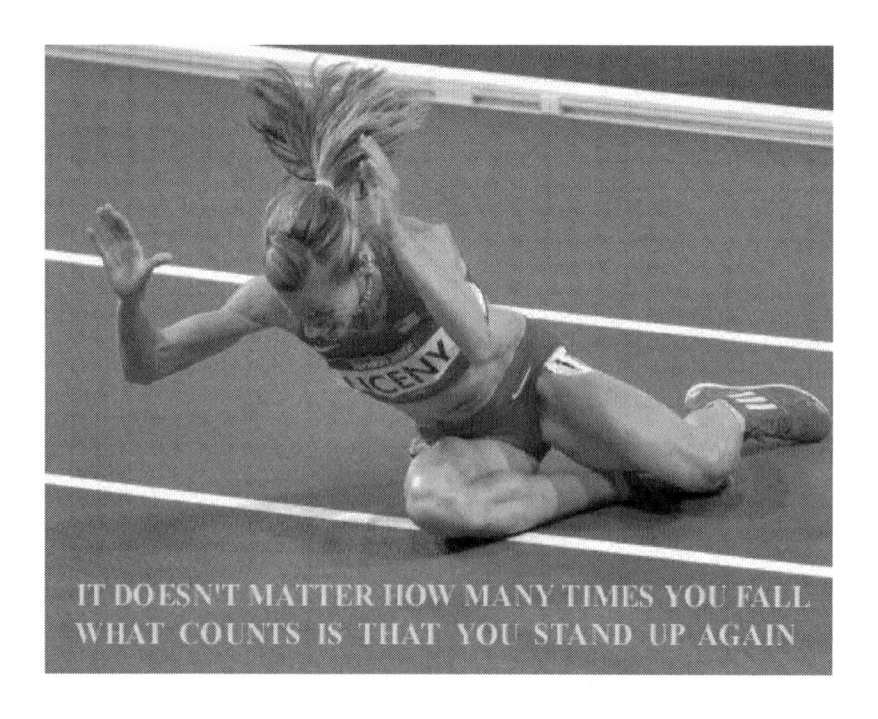

IT DOESN'T MATTER HOW MANY TIMES YOU FALL
WHAT COUNTS IS THAT YOU STAND UP AGAIN

Sources:

http://www.psychologytoday.com/blog/the-blame-game/201205/throw-away-your-vision-board-0

http://sunshineimpressions.wordpress.com/2013/02/17/visual-action-board/

http://buzn1029.cbslocal.com/2012/12/31/stall-secrets-turn-your-vision-board-into-an-action-board-for-2013/

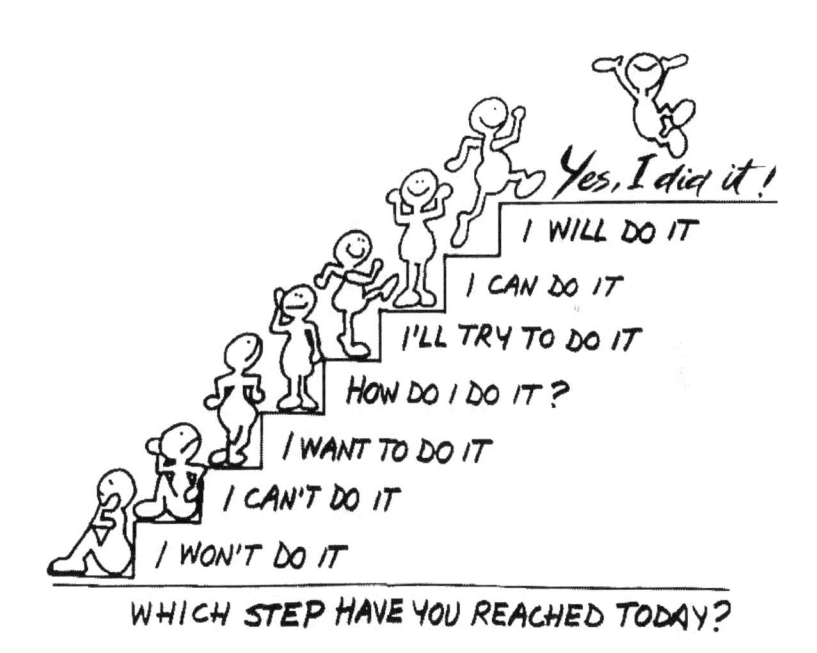

Yes, I did it!
I WILL DO IT
I CAN DO IT
I'LL TRY TO DO IT
HOW DO I DO IT?
I WANT TO DO IT
I CAN'T DO IT
I WON'T DO IT

WHICH STEP HAVE YOU REACHED TODAY?

15. Powerful Words Evoke Powerful Images

15.1 The Power of Metaphors

by Enrique Montiel

Some words evoke strong images. They allow us to send out messages which trigger the visualization power of our readers and listeners.

"The metaphor is perhaps one of man's most fruitful potentialities. It's efficacy verges on magic. It seems a tool for creation which God forgot inside one of His creatures when He made him."

(José Ortegay Gasset - 1925, p. 35)

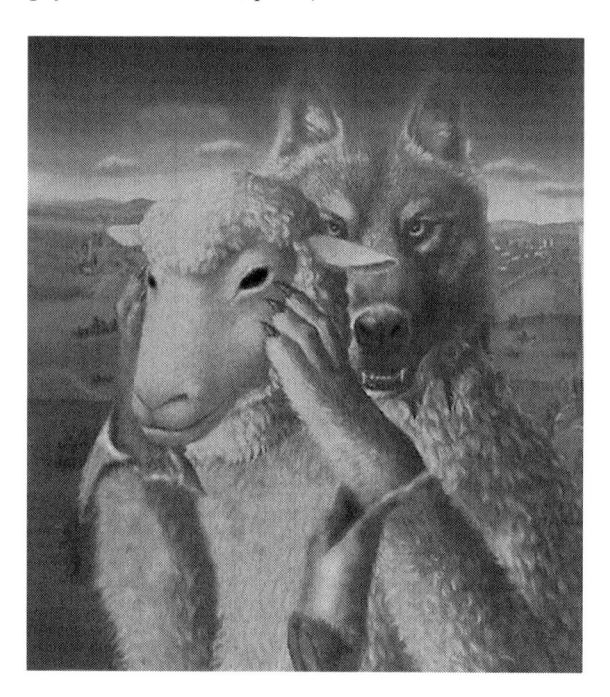

Have you ever wondered what people mean when they say "I can see light at the end of the tunnel", or "I feel like I've hit a brick wall"?

Metaphors are often used as a way of expressing views that may be difficult to describe literally or may be too challenging to state as they are. They deserve your attention because they are giving new messages at more than one level of feelings, values and another person's experience of the situation..

What are your beliefs about life?

If you answer the question, "What are your beliefs about life?", your answer will probably come in the form of a metaphor. Amongst the many possible answers are life is an adventure, a struggle, a war zone, a dress rehearsal, the main act, a competition, a dance or possibly even a game.

As human beings, we constantly think and speak in metaphors. Often people talk of "being caught between a rock and a hard place." They feel like they're "struggling to keep their head above water" because "they're carrying the world on their shoulders." Do you think you might be at least a little bit stressed out if you thought about dealing with your life challenges in terms of "struggling to keep your head above water" rather than "opportunities to become emotionally wealthier"?

15.2 What is a metaphor?

Analogy, simile and Metaphor

In analogy, parts of B may be compared with parts of A, but B is not considered to be the same as A. The association is much weaker than is the case in similes or metaphors.

Examples:

Analogy: People may treat the world as their stage

Similes: are constrained in that the word 'like' or 'as' is explicitly used.

Similes: The world is like a stage, he's strong as a bear, he's as big as a mountain, she's as dark as the night, she's fresh as the morning dew,

Metaphors basically say 'A is B', unlike similes which say 'A is like B' and analogies which offer a vaguer linkage between A and B.

This gives a stronger association between A and B in metaphor. B is effectively overlaid and A, and everything about B is attributed to A. Thus A effectively becomes B.

Metaphors: All the world's a stage, I am the good shepherd, I am the Son of God, I am the lamb of God, you are the sun of my life, you are the air that I breathe, she's a black crow,

15.3 List of strong metaphors

- A heart of stone (from Rebecca)
- He has the heart of a lion
- You are the sun in my sky
- You are the light in my life
- She is my East and my West, my compass.
- You had better pull your socks up
- Life is a mere dream, a fleeting shadow on a cloudy day.
- Love is a lemon - either bitter of sweet (from Scott)
- Drowning in the sea
- Jumping for joy
- Rolling in dough
- Apple of my eye

- It is raining cats and dogs
- Love is a fragile flower opening to the warmth of Spring
- Information travels faster in this modern age as our days start crawling away.
- Life has a tendency to come back and bite you in the ass.
- A riverboat shall be my horse.
- A light in a sea of darkness.
- Strength and dignity are her clothing.
- A laugh in a sea of sadness.
- The noise is music to my ears
- He swam in the sea of diamonds
- His belt was a snake curling around his waist
- Love is a camera, full of memories.
- She ran like the Wind
- Love is a growing garland.
- Your friendship is the picture to my frame
- Authority is a chair, it needs legs to stand up.
- Once your hearts been broken it grows back bigger.
- His hair is a white snowflake and his hair is a messy haystack
- You are the expression of my heart. You care for me and love me all the time.
- I'm Heartbroken
- The pigeons fountained into the air
- His hair was bone white
- He tried to help but his legs were rubber
- It's raining men
- Kicked the bucket
- The sea is a hungry dog.
- She is a dog when she eats
- He has a voice of a wolf.
- Crocodiles' teeth are white daggers.
- Apple of my heart
- A roundabout is a turtle shell.
- Fire is day, when it goes out it's night
- School is a gateway to adulthood

- He slithered into town quietly so no one would notice when he dug his fangs in and slowly poisoned their minds.
- Leaping with laughter - (Trinita)
- The silence was a blood-cuddling scream of anguish, set out to break my soul (Kiwi)
- The Big Bang. (Fred Hoyle)
- All the world's a stage, and all the men and women merely players. They have their exits and their entrances. (William Shakespeare)
- Art washes away from the soul the dust of everyday life. (Pablo Picasso)
- I am the good shepherd, ... and I lay down my life for the sheep. (The Bible, John 10:14-15)
- All religions, arts and sciences are branches of the same tree. (Albert Einstein)
- Chaos is a friend of mine. (Bob Dylan)
- All our words are but crumbs that fall down from the feast of the mind. (Khalil Gibran)
- If you want a love message to be heard, it has got to be sent out. To keep a lamp burning, we have to keep putting oil in it. (Mother Teresa)
- America has tossed its cap over the wall of space. (John F. Kennedy)
- A hospital bed is a parked taxi with the meter running. (Groucho Marx)
- A good conscience is a continual Christmas. (Benjamin Franklin)
- Let us be grateful to people who make us happy, they are the charming gardeners who make our souls blossom. (Marcel Proust)
- And your very flesh shall be a great poem. (Walt Whitman)
- Advertising is the rattling of a stick inside a swill bucket. (George Orwell)
- Dying is a wild night and a new road. (Emily Dickinson)
- Fill your paper with the breathings of your heart. (William Wordsworth)
- Conscience is a man's compass.(Vincent Van Gogh)

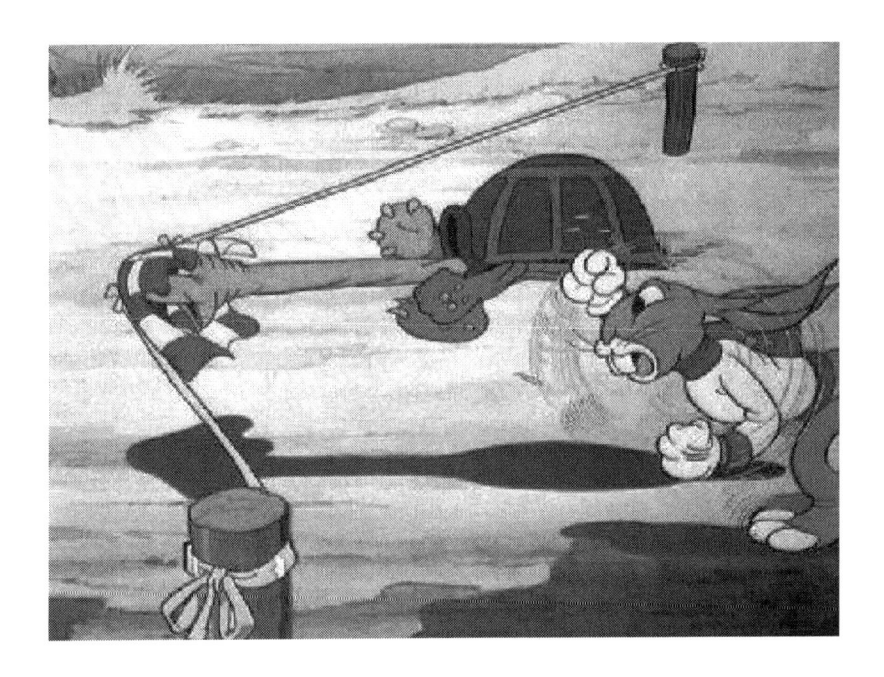

15.4 The power of metaphors

If I say 'You look like a dog', then I am placing some of the visual attributes of a dog on you. If, however, I say 'you are a dog', then I am saying that you are a dog in all ways, and that all attributes that a dog has, you have.

Metaphors are thus much stronger than similes or analogies, as the vehicle holds more weight than the subject that it replaces.

The power of metaphors is in the way that they change the subject by bringing new thinking and ideas, extending and changing the way that a person thinks about something.

15.5 Limitations of metaphors

The power and the limitation of the metaphor is the way that the vehicle brings not just a little bit of understanding but a whole world. When you say 'I am a dog', you bring the entire world of dogginess to the subject.

The underlying assumption is that the vehicle is correct and that in any conflict of meaning, the subject is wrong.

This can be a limitation and a trap, as you may want to bring some attributes but not some of the less desirable ones. Metaphors must thus be used with care. If I say 'you are stupid', then 'stupid' effectively replaces 'you', and all of you becomes all of stupid.

15.6 Metaphor is how we learn

Metaphor is one of the primary ways in which we learn. Learning is the process of making new associations in our minds, creating meanings, and metaphors are ideally suited for this. Most simply it is communicating or explaining a concept by likening it to something else. The two things may have little actual resemblance to each other, but our familiarity with one allows us to gain understanding of the other.

Metaphors can empower us by expanding and enriching our experience of life. However, having only one metaphor to describe your total experience is a great way to limit your life. Just imagine only paying attention to a single colour hue of a perfect rainbow.

With all the power that metaphors wield over our lives, the scary part is that most of us have never consciously selected the metaphors with which we use to represent things to ourselves. As a result of this many people have metaphors that greatly help them in their professions, but create challenges at home; the attorney that cross examines his or her spouse at home every night.

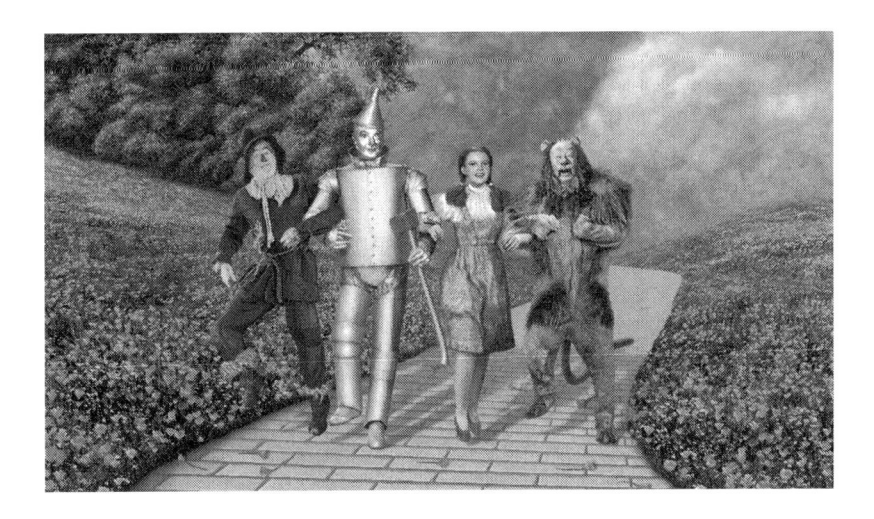

15.7 Where did you get your metaphors?

You picked them up from the environment around you, from your parents, teachers, co-workers, friends, literature, music, television and film. Chances are you didn't think about their impact, or maybe you didn't even think about them at all, and then they just became habits. We naturally adopt metaphors out of our need to place meaning to the world around us. Unfortunately, though, by not paying attention to the metaphors we adopt we often are disempowered by the limiting beliefs that come with them. And few things are more debilitating than toxic metaphors.

For some people, "life is like playing a game or a sport." How might that colour your perceptions? It might make life fun! It might make it somewhat competitive. It might be a chance for you to play and enjoy the one short life you have a lot more. Some people say, "If it's a game , then there are going to be losers." Other people ask, "What rules can we set up so that everybody wins?" It all depends on what beliefs you've decided to attach to the word "game".

Can you see how changing just one significant metaphor could instantly change your experience of life instantly?

This is an example of what's called a pivot point, a global change, where just making this one change would transform the way you think and feel in multiple areas of your life.

15.8 Test this out for yourself. Your exercise:

1. Answer the question, "Life is like" (Write down the metaphors you've already chosen for yourself),

2. Create new, more empowering metaphors to replace the one's you've written down by asking yourself, "If life was like playing a win win sport it would be".,

3. Decide that you are going to live with these new, empowering metaphors for the next thirty days.

Take control of your metaphors now and create a new world of possibility, richness, wonder, joy and fulfilment. "Life is painting a picture, not doing a sum." - Oliver Wendell Holmes, Jr.

How we think, how we make sense of the universe, is by means of metaphors (Beckett, 2003; Turbayne, 1962).

Metaphors are not just a literary flourish used by those with a poetic turn of mind, but a fundamental tool that has been used by humans from the earliest times to shape thought and action (Lakoff & Johnson, 2003). Metaphors are so pervasive and embedded in the way we think about things that we often don't even recognize when we have used them

Metaphors function positively and negatively. They have the power to help us create meaning and understanding and to improve how we lead.They also have the power to manipulate, to shut down thinking, to deflect creativity, and to harm. Their very ubiquity, their indispensableness, lends metaphors great power.

15.9 How metaphors work

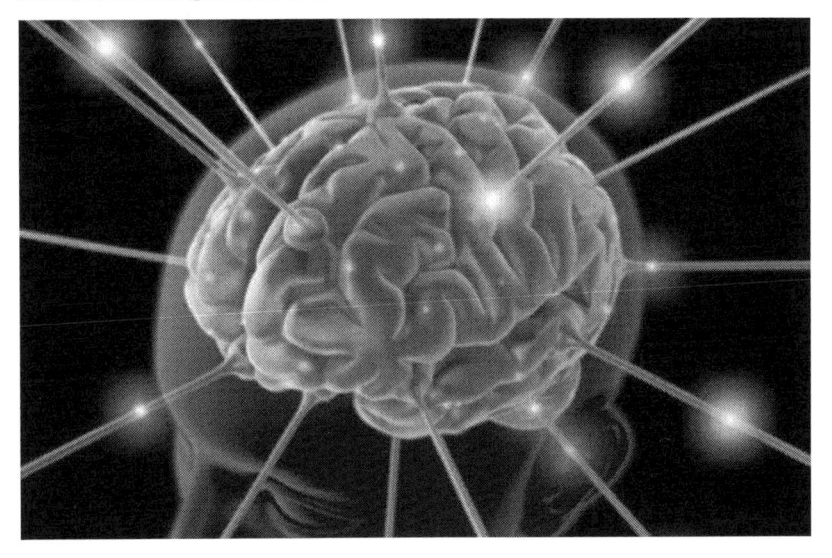

To fully understand the power of metaphors we need to know how they work.

1. The first phenomenon of metaphors is that they trigger an effect (Camp, 2005).

By comparing two things that are both similar and dissimilar, they throw the reader or listener into a state of momentary uncertainty, where the degree and significance of the similarity and dissimilarity must be considered. We are tilted off balance and find ourselves "exiles from the familiar" (Burns, 1972, p. 109).

The term used to capture this mental state is "liminality," defined by Anderson (2005) as "the ambiguous condition of being between, at the limits of existing structures and where new structures are emerging ... a transformative stage where a thing is in process of becoming something else" (pp. 590–591).

A metaphor takes us into a state of liminality, where we work at creating sense: "It pre-empts our attention and propels us on a quest for the underlying truth. We are launched into a creative, inventive, pleasurable act" (Swanson, 1979, p. 162). The effect is greatest when the similarity is perceived to be not total but significant, so that meaning is created.

For example, Barack Obama's generation is now described as "Generation Jones" instead of the "late baby boomers." Wells (2009) indicates that "Generation Jones" reflects the "yearning (or 'jonesing') of its members for the coolness of the 1960s and their parents' efforts to keep up with the Joneses" (p. 36).

2. The second aspect of the use of metaphor is that it constructs a relationship between the user and the receiver.

Cohen (1979) believes that by using a metaphor the writer or speaker extends a kind of invitation. To respond, the reader or listener must actively engage and, by doing so, a degree of connection and, to Cohen, empathy and trust, is created. Such trust has the potential to be a positive or negative in creating acuity in the receiver. For example, Schapper's (2009) title, "Investing in a Girl's Education is Like Watering a Neighbour's Tree" invites the reader to consider in what ways watering the tree of a neighbour might be like the education of a girl, but not a boy. The reader has to create his or her own sense, imagining first what the attitude might be of someone watering a plant that belongs to another: generosity, foolishness, a community gesture toward the future?

Then there is consideration of the tree belonging to someone. Does this mean that the girl belongs to someone in the way that a tree might?

We have only touched the surface of the rich meanings, the sense making, the challenge to one's values created by this one image. The reader cannot receive it passively. He or she must actively draw on personal experience to make judgments in response and thereby be drawn into a relationship with the writer to learn more.

Engagement with metaphors has the potential to sharpen analytical acuity, to create new ideas, and to demand an active process of meaning making to understand what people do or how they relate to each other.

However, metaphors do not always work in this way. Some metaphors have become so embedded in our language and thinking that they do not trigger the effect just described. Instead, they have become "dead" or "frozen" (Goodwin, 1996; Tsoukas, 1991). Cornelissen (2002) defines dead metaphors as those concepts which have become so familiar and so habitual in our theoretical vocabulary that not only have we ceased to be aware of their metaphorical precepts, but also have we stopped to ascribe such qualities, instead we take them as "literal terms." (p. 261)

When educators speak of "delivering" programs, or of "strategy," they are not generally aware that they are using metaphors. For example, in a speech by the former UK prime minister, Tony Blair (2005), outlining reforms that "will create and sustain irreversible change for the better in schools" he uses such metaphors as:

"Over the last 50 years, state education has improved.
And that improvement has ACCELERATED in the last eight years.
But successive reforms since the war have not always DELIVERED all that they aimed to DELIVER.
What is different this time is that we have learned what works.
We have the experience of SUCCESSFUL schools.
What we must see now is a system of independent state schools, underpinned by fair admissions and fair funding, where parents are equipped and enabled to DRIVE improvement, driven by the aspirations of parents."

The metaphors indicated here by us in capital letters are likely to be taken as literal by most. That is, listeners to the speech will not consciously engage with assessing the degree of similarity and dissimilarity and its significance.

However, the message of central government and parents acting rather as machines, accelerating speed, delivering what is intended, driving, is evident once pointed out. It is schools and teachers who are to be driven and accelerated. The machine metaphor establishes education as a thing, not as people. While the metaphors may be dead in the sense of not registering as metaphors, they are very much alive in reflecting a worldview of education, a cultural and historical position. Dead metaphors have the capacity to shape thinking and values as much as those that are live.

15.10 How metaphors influence

Researchers wanting to understand how metaphors shape the way people think about things, have found that different metaphors don't just make people think of different solutions, but of which solution is best ("Mind the power of metaphors: study" - Times LIVE | 30 January, 2013 11:44)

The research, published in PloS One, follows another study in which researchers had people come up with solutions to crime, where in one metaphor it was compared to a virus and another to a beast.

In that study what they found was that when crime was described as a beast people tended to argue for catching criminals and subjecting them to harsher punishments.

When crime was described as a virus, people suggested tackling root causes such as poverty, or educational reforms.

The new study was thus begun to see how metaphors influenced which solutions people tended to pick.

They set up a set of four experiments to test the power of the two metaphors once more, but this time gave them a series of possible reforms to tackle those issues. What they found was that they did indeed change which solutions people favoured.

"People who read that crime was a beast were more likely to rank one of the enforcement-oriented responses as the best (42%) than those who read that crime was a virus (31%)," the researchers wrote.

Not only that, but most people did not include the metaphor when selecting what motivated their response, writing "we found that people rarely identified the metaphor as influential in their thinking despite its influence. We found that the metaphors influenced even those people who could not remember the metaphorical frame."

The researchers concluded that study reveals that people can be unwittingly swayed by metaphors when reasoning about social policy. Metaphors encourage particular conceptualisations of problems and, depending on the situation, can be helpful or misleading. We hope that coming to appreciate the role that metaphors play in reasoning can help decision-makers be mindful of the limitations and the virtues of the metaphors they chose to frame issues. .

15.11 Powerful Metaphor Communication

In our modern, western world the tradition of telling and listening to stories has been replaced with passive activities of watching television or playing computer games which do little to generate connections for change in the brain. The most powerful communicators of our time such as, Nelson Mandela, Winston Churchill, or Martin Luther King all used metaphor and anecdote as a way of connecting with people and putting across their message in ways that many thousands were able to understand and appreciate. Many other professionals, experts in their respective fields of psychotherapy and psychology including Gregory Bateson and

Milton Erickson used a variety of metaphorical approaches in their work.

There is no doubt that metaphor works at different levels. The conscious mind processes the content of a story while the unconscious mind is receiving the hidden or embedded messages sprinkled throughout the story. The embedded messages create the possibility of generative change, while the conscious mind focuses on the surface level of the story. Expert story tellers create parallel realities in the story as often happens in dreams so that people at the unconscious level can resolve their inner difficulties painlessly and without feeling threatened.

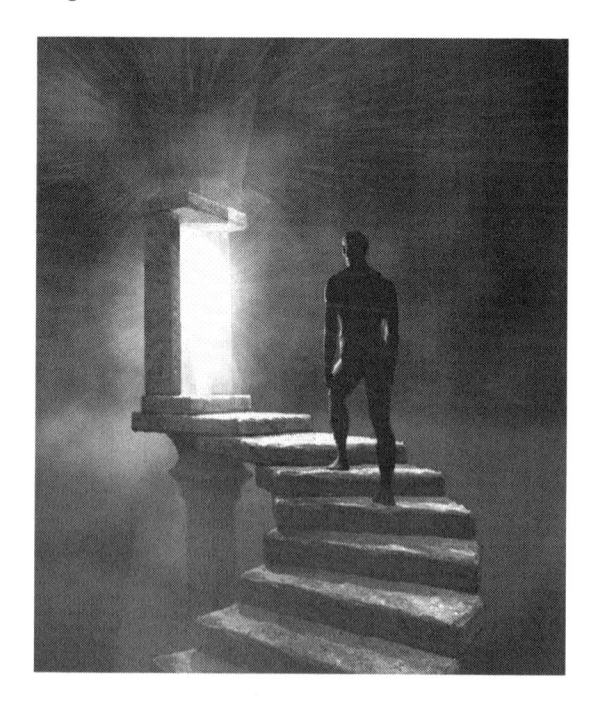

15.12 The Metaphor of our lives:

We are continuously telling ourselves different versions of our life story. The inner voice whispers and sometimes shouts the script. We are often quite good at reciting the age old story of how hard we have struggled to overcome our perceived problems. These self-constructed versions of our life script are simply personal metaphors and not necessarily true or accurate. These stories unconsciously guide and deeply influence our perceptions and behaviour in the face of life experiences.

Meta-learning Solutions help you investigate your own stories and when uncovered facilitate you to explore how different processes for modifying or even replacing with new stories will serve you more effectively in the future.

Sources:

Fenwick W. English recently co-authored, with Jacky Lumby, the book, "Leadership as lunacy: And other metaphors for educational leadership". Published by Corwin Press,

Enrique Montiel is a researcher and developer of life enhancement systems. He is the inventor of LBD, EBD, and CBD technologies which he promotes in his private practice and through his company, Life Enhancement Systems. Enrique is also a published writer, accomplished independent filmmaker and Olympic hopeful.

Enrique Montiel is a San Diego, California native residing in Colorado Springs, Colorado where he is currently conducting peak performance and achievement research as well as speaking and facilitating his personal and professional development programs throughout the United States. He can be reached at enrique@enriquemontiel.com, 719 227-7177, www.enriquemontiel.com

http://www.meta-learning.co.uk/index.php/advice/entry/the_power_of_metaphor/

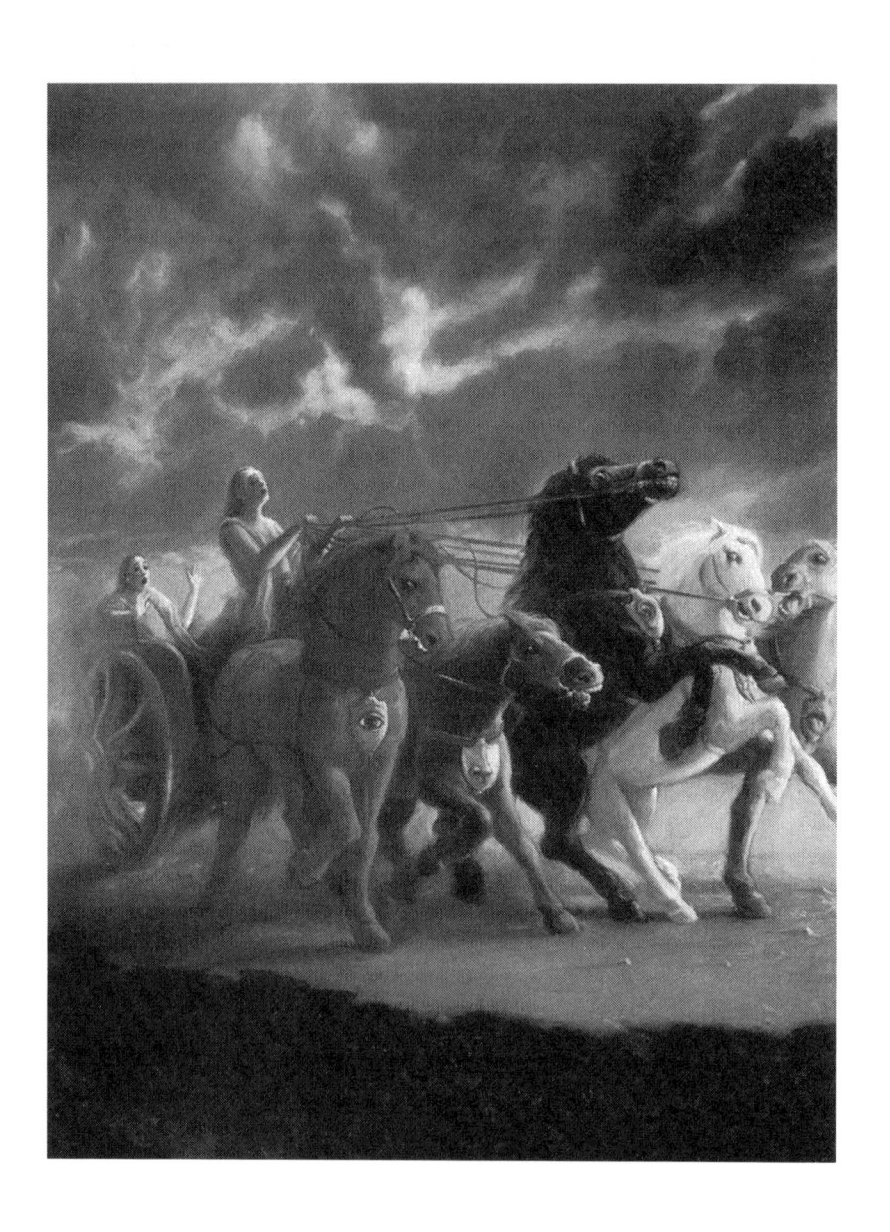

16. The Bucket List

"Every man dies – Not every man really lives." ~ William Ross

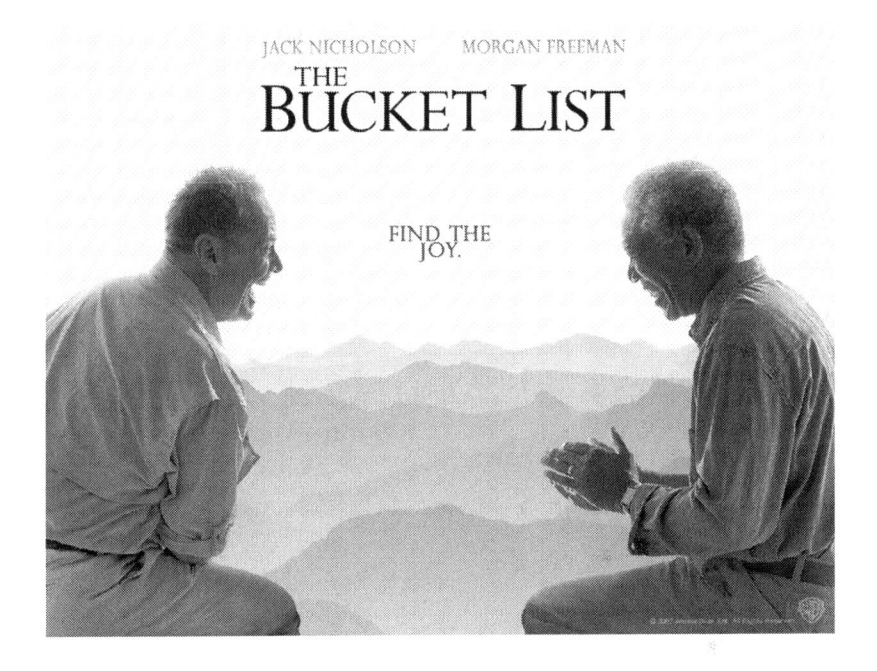

16.1 What is a Bucket List?

bucket list: a list of all the goals you want to achieve, dreams you want to fulfil and life experiences you desire to experience before you die.

Etymology: Derived from kick the bucket ("to die") + list; hence "list of things to do before you die".

Apparently coined for the 2007 film The Bucket List; articles about the movie are the earliest known uses.

In "The Bucket List" two terminally ill men escape from a cancer ward and head off on a road trip with a wish list, a "bucket list", of to-dos before they die.

The essence of any good bucket list consists of overcoming fears, achieving goals, realizing dreams and enjoy simple pleasures.

Whether it's an exotic adventure half-way around the world or something simpler, like spending more time with your family or friends, what matters is that you experience all the good and phenomenal things earth offers.

16.2 Why Create A Bucket List? (from Celes)

If you don't live your days by personal goals and plans, chances are you spend most of your time caught up in a flurry of day-to-day activities. Ever feel your days are passing you by without any tangible output to speak of? What did you accomplish in the past 3 months? What are your upcoming goals for the next 3 months? Look at the things you did and the things you're planning to do next – Do they mean anything to you if you are to die today? Having a bucket list reminds you of what's really important so you can act on them.

Even if you frequently live by goals or to-do lists, they are probably framed within a certain social context e.g. performance, career, health. A bucket list opens up the context. It's a forum to set anything and everything you've ever wanted to do, whether it's big, small or random.

It's just like planning ahead all the highlights you want for YOUR whole life. Even though goal setting is already my staple activity, I still found many new things to do while I was writing on my bucket list. It was an incredibly insightful exercise. What's more, coming up with my list gave me a whole new layer of enthusiasm knowing what's in store ahead!

The objective of creating a bucket list isn't to instil some kind of a race against time or to create aversion toward death. I don't see our existence to be limited to just our physical years on earth – I don't see our existence to be limited to just our physical years on earth – our physical lifespan is but a short speck of our existence in the universe.

The whole point of creating your list is to maximize every moment of our existence and live our life to the fullest. It's a reminder of all the things we want to achieve in our time here, so that instead of pandering our time in pointless activities, we are directing it fully toward what matters to us.

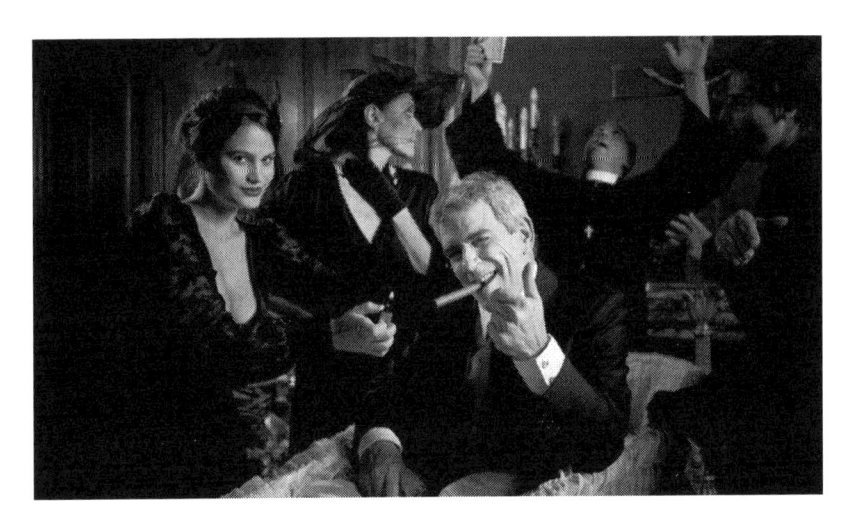

16.3 How to Create Your Bucket List

If you don't have a bucket list, I highly recommend you to create one.

- ➢ How much does it cost? Zero.
- ➢ How long does it take? Probably 30 minutes to an hour, or more

> What do you stand to gain? Significant clarity and focus on what you want from your life.

It's an invaluable exchange.

If you have already written your bucket list before, take this opportunity to review it. See if there are new items you want to add-on. If so, add them in. Check if all the items listed are still relevant. If not, remove them.

Now, take out your pen and paper or open up a text document.

Start writing down what comes to mind as you read these questions:
- What if you were to die tomorrow?
- What would you wish you could do before you die?
- What would you do if you had unlimited time, money and resources?
- What have you always wanted to do but have not done yet?
- Any countries, places or locations you want to visit?
- What are your biggest goals and dreams?
- What do you want to see in person?
- What achievements do you want to have?
- What experiences do you want to have / feel?
- Are there any special moments you want to witness?
- What activities or skills do you want to learn or try out?
- What are the most important things you can ever do?
- What would you like to say/do together with other people? People you love? Family? Friends?
- Are there any specific people you want to meet in person?
- What do you want to achieve in the different areas: Social, Love, Family, Career, Finance, Health (Your weight, Fitness level), Spiritual?
- What do you need to do to lead a life of the greatest meaning?

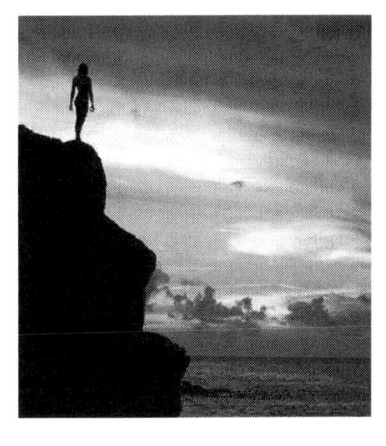

Come up with as many items as you can. The items should be things you have not done yet. Don't stop until you finish listing at least 101 things!

If you find yourself stuck, chances are you are mentally limiting/constraining yourself. Release those shackles – Your bucket list is meant to be a list of everything you want to achieve, do, see, feel and experience in your life.

16.4 101 items to consider for your bucket list.

Some of the items might spark off your inspiration for other things too!

- ✓ Travel all around the world
- ✓ Visit all the countries in the world
- ✓ Visit all the Wonders of the World
- ✓ Go on a road trip
- ✓ Visit a castle in England
- ✓ Watch cherry blossoms in Japan
- ✓ See the Mona Lisa in Louvre (Paris)
- ✓ Go backpacking across at least 10 locations
- ✓ Pack your bags and set off for a random location with no itinerary planned at all
- ✓ Go swimming with dolphins
- ✓ Live in a different country for at least 6 months
- ✓ Go deep into the heart of Mother Nature: Go trekking in a rainforest; Camp out in the wilds; Walk in a valley; Visit a waterfall; Swim in an ocean; Walk in a valley
- ✓ Experience marine life up close
- ✓ See snow (if you haven't before)

- ✓ Learn a new language
- ✓ Visit a volcano
- ✓ Fly in a helicopter
- ✓ Go on a cruise in the sea
- ✓ See the Northern Lights
- ✓ Experience a sunset
- ✓ Experience a sunrise
- ✓ Witness a solar eclipse
- ✓ Fall asleep on grassy plains
- ✓ Go stargazing
- ✓ Fly in a hot-air balloon across a country

- ✓ Run a marathon
- ✓ Take part in a triathlon
- ✓ Take up a new sport.
  Some examples:
- ✓ Technique sports: Archery, Golf, Bowling, Billiard, Skateboarding, Skating, Roller-blading, Ice skating,
- ✓ Water sports: Water rafting, Kayaking, Wakeboarding, Sailing, Scuba diving, Snorkelling, Swimming,
- ✓ Group sports: Soccer, Rugby, Baseball, Basketball, Ultimate Frisbee
- ✓ Racket sports: Squash, Badminton, Tennis, Table tennis
- ✓ Extreme sports: Bungee jumping, Skydiving, Parachuting, Paragliding, Ice climbing
- ✓ Go skiing
- ✓ Learn horseback riding
- ✓ Learn a strategy game
- ✓ Climb a mountain
- ✓ Learn a martial art

- ✓ Write a letter to at least 3 of your closest friends to let them know how much they mean to you
- ✓ Perform a kind deed to at least 5 strangers without expecting anything in return

- ✓ Make friends with at least 5 strangers on the street
- ✓ Bury the hatchet with all the enemies / people you had conflict with in the past or now
- ✓ Call the customer service (of a service provider you like) just to thank them for the great service.
- ✓ Tell your parents (and siblings too if you have them) that you love them.
- ✓ Connect with the teachers from your past – college, high school, junior high, all of it. Let them know how they have shaped your life.
- ✓ Identify someone who has inspired you the most in your life. Let him/her know how much he/she has inspired you
- ✓ Be a mentor to someone
- ✓ Give a heartfelt surprise to someone
- ✓ Volunteer at a hospice
- ✓ Change the world
- ✓ Help someone in need
- ✓ Make a difference in someone's life
- ✓ Offer your service to a humanitarian cause

- ✓ Resign from a job you don't like
- ✓ Try out a new profession in a different field
- ✓ Pursue your passion
- ✓ Start your own business doing something you love
- ✓ Achieve financial abundance with your passion
- ✓ Write a book on something that means a lot to you
- ✓ Sing your favourite song to an audience
- ✓ Do public speaking in front of 10,000 people
- ✓ Plant your own tree and watch it grow
- ✓ Own a pet (or more if you desire!): dog, cat, rabbit, hamster, tortoise, fish, snake, frog, etc
- ✓ Throw a mega party
- ✓ Get a complete makeover (change everything, from your hair style, hair colour, image, clothes) and get a different look: one which you would never have thought of trying!

- ✓ Achieve your ideal weight.
- ✓ Learn wine appreciation
- ✓ Join a social etiquette class and further refine your mannerisms

- ✓ Be a matchmaker: Introduce your single friends to each other (the rest is up to them!)
- ✓ Go on a blind date! (for the singles!)
- ✓ Fall in love
- ✓ Be in love!
- ✓ Get on a romantic getaway

- ✓ Go for future education in a different specialization
- ✓ Play a (new) musical instrument: Piano, Violin, Harmonica, Flute, Guitar, Drum, Trumpet
- ✓ Win a lucky draw
- ✓ Take up dancing: Salsa, Line dance, Tap dance, Tango, Ballroom dancing, etc
- ✓ Act in a film (self production or otherwise)
- ✓ Get featured on TV/radio/print/newspapers for an achievement you are proud of
- ✓ Knit a scarf
- ✓ Create your dream home (Read: Does Your Room Inspire You?)
- ✓ Whip up the best meal ever for your loved ones
- ✓ Bake a cake for someone special
- ✓ Live through 4 seasons of the year – Spring, summer, autumn, winter
- ✓ Read a book on a subject you'd never have thought of reading
- ✓ Fly a kite
- ✓ If you are a non-vegetarian, try out vegetarianism for 21 days and experience it for yourself - After that, try veganism - Followed by raw veganism. Then conclude which is the best diet for you.

- ✓ Fold a 1,000 origami cranes and give them to someone special
- ✓ Conquer your biggest fear
- ✓ Tell at least 10 people about your bucket list and encourage them to do the same
- ✓ Go on a meditation retreat
- ✓ Experience an OBE (out of body experience)
- ✓ Start a social movement on a cause you believe in
- ✓ Get closure on all your hurt, grievances and unhappiness of the past
- ✓ Organize a picnic outing
- ✓ Do something completely crazy and out of character
- ✓ Fly first class
- ✓ Hit bulls eye on a dartboard
- ✓ Have dinner with someone you had only dreamed of meeting
- ✓ Ride a roller coaster
- ✓ Try out front-line customer service jobs such being a waiter/waitress for a month just for the experience
- ✓ Do a somersault
- ✓ Learn sign language
- ✓ Go to a costume party and dress up as your fantasy character
- ✓ Gain enlightenment

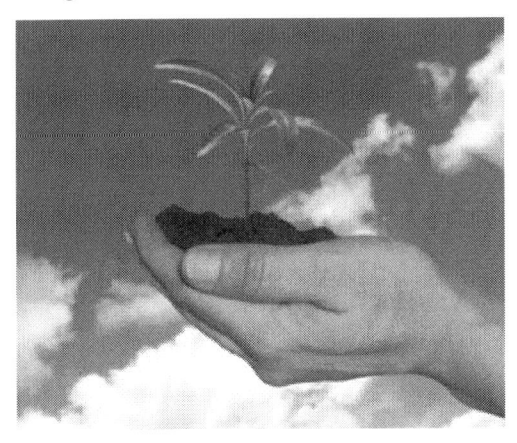

Get Into Action!

16.5 After you finish your list:

Here is what to do next

Start acting on them! Plan out the successful path toward these goals – For this, read my 7-part Successful Goal Achievement series.

Be reminded of the list all the time. Use environmental reinforcement – put them up in a prominent spot where you will see them every day / very regularly. Put it in your life handbook, set it as your wallpaper, pin it on your notice board, print it out, stick it on your wardrobe/locker.

Share them with your family and friends. Inspire them to create their own bucket lists too! This way, you also create accountability for yourself as you complete the items on your list.

Don't limit your bucket list items to a certain definition. Sometimes opportunity present itself in a totally different manner. Keep your eyes peeled! The universe will start throwing things your way.

Review your list regularly. Cross out the things after you do them. See if some of the items become irrelevant and if there are new things you want to add. Just as you finish the items, you'll add new ones as they come along. There is absolutely no reason why your list should ever be empty. There is such an incredible wealth of things, events, activities, experiences to witness/go through in life that it's impossible that you will ever be done with living. Likewise for me, I'm continuously completing and adding on new items that will help me live my life to the fullest, so my bucket list always has new items to accomplish.

Sources:

http://personalexcellence.co/blog/whats-on-your-bucket-list-101-things-to-do-before-you-die/

On Lifed.com you'll find 225 things to do before you die. Check them all at   http://www.lifed.com/bucket-list-225-things-to-do-before-you-die

Catalog all the stuf you want to accomplish before you expire is a great way to visualize what is really important to you! You may find inspiration for your list at: http://bucketlist.org

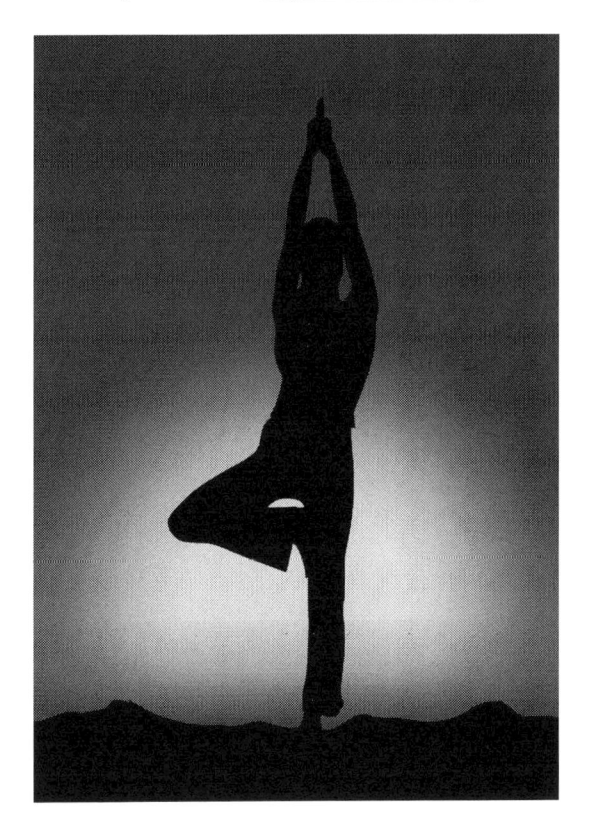

17. The Power of Mental Imagery

The Project Gutenberg EBook of Power of Mental Imagery

This eBook is for the use of anyone anywhere at no cost and with almost no restrictions whatsoever. You may copy it, give it away or re-use it under the terms of the Project Gutenberg License included with this eBook or online at www.gutenberg.org

Produced by David Clarke, Suzan Flanagan and the Online Distributed Proofreading Team at http://www.pgdp.net (This file was produced from images generously made available by The Internet Archive/Million Book Project)

Applied Psychology

POWER OF MENTAL IMAGERY

BY WARREN HILTON, A.B., L.L.B.

FOUNDER OF THE SOCIETY OF APPLIED PSYCHOLOGY

ISSUED UNDER THE AUSPICES OF

THE LITERARY DIGEST

FOR THE SOCIETY OF APPLIED PSYCHOLOGY

NEW YORK AND LONDON
1920

COPYRIGHT 1914
BY THE APPLIED PSYCHOLOGY PRESS
SAN FRANCISCO

17.1 HOW TO INFLUENCE OTHERS THROUGH MENTAL IMAGERY (CHAPTER III)

A Rule for Influencing Others

THE practical importance of the fact of mental imagery and of the individual differences in power of mental imagery is very great. They should be particularly taken into account in any business or profession in which one seeks to implant knowledge or conviction in the mind of another.

Application to Pedagogy

The underlying principle in such cases is this: *To the mind you are seeking to convince or educate, present your facts in as many different ways and as realistically as possible, so that there may be a variety of images, each serving as a clue to prompt the memory.*

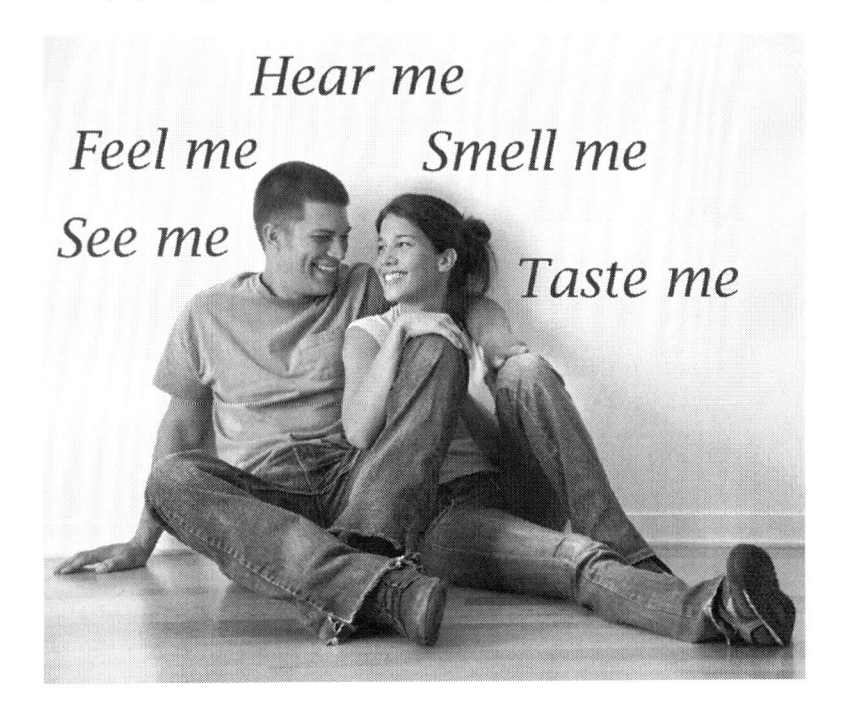

Hear me
Feel me   *Smell me*
See me
              Taste me

We cannot do more at this point than indicate a few minor phases of the practical application of the principles of mental imagery.

In the old days geography was taught simply with a book and maps. Today children also use their hands in moulding relief maps in sand or clay, and mountains and rivers have acquired a meaning they never had before.

In the days of the oral "spelling match" boys and girls were better spellers than products of a later school system, because they used not only the eye to see the printed word, the arm and hand to feel in writing it, but also the ear to hear it and the vocal muscles to utter it. And because of this fact oral spelling is being brought back to the schoolroom.

How to Sell Goods by Mental Imagery

If you have pianos to advertise, do not limit your advertisement to a beautiful picture of the mahogany case and general words telling the reader that it is "the best." Pianos are musical instruments, and the descriptive words should first of all call up delightful *auditory images* in your reader's mind.

If you have for sale an article of food, do not simply tell your customer how good it is. Let him see it, feel it, and particularly *taste it*, if you want him to call for it the next time he enters your store.

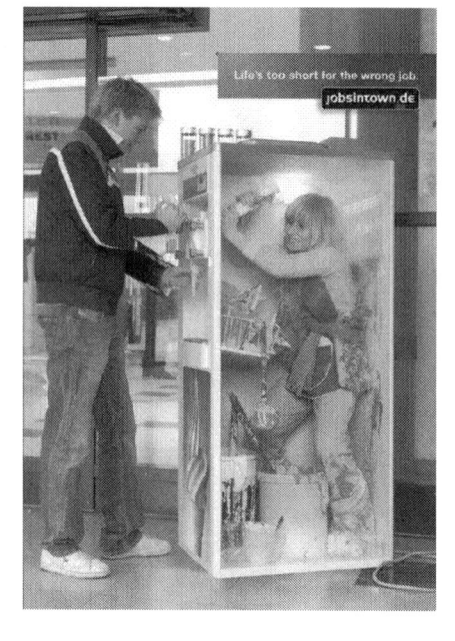

248

A Study of Advertisements

Turn, for example, to the advertisement of a certain brand of chocolate (ad deleted, shows girl serving chocolate)), facing. The daintily spread table, the pretty girl, the steaming cup, the evident satisfaction of the man, who looks accustomed to good living,— these elements combine in a skilful appeal to the senses. Turn now to another advertisement of this same brand of chocolate, shown facing (ad also deleted – shows machinery). The purpose here is to inform you as to the large quantity of cocoa beans roasted in the company's furnaces. Whether this fact is of any consequence or not, the impression you get from the picture is of a wheelbarrow full of something that looks like coal being trundled by a dirty workman, while the shovel by the furnace door and the cocoa beans scattered about the floor remind one of a begrimed iron foundry.

The Words that Create Desire

The only words that will ever sell anything *are graphic words, picturesque words, words that call up distinct and definite mental pictures of an attractive kind.*

The more sensory images we have of any object the better we know it.

If you want to make a first impression lasting, make it vivid. It will then photograph itself upon the memory and arouse the curiosity.

A boy who is a poor visualizer will never make a good artist. A man who is a poor visualizer is out of place as a photographer or a picture salesman.

A Key for Selecting a Calling

No person with weak auditory images should follow music as a profession or attempt to sell phonographs or musical instruments or become a telephone or telegraph operator or stenographer.

No man who can but faintly imagine the taste of things should try to write advertisements for articles of food.

Remember the rule: *To the mind you are seeking to convince or educate present your facts in as many different ways and as realistically as possible, so that there may be a variety of images, each serving as a clue to prompt the memory.*

You can put this rule to practical use at once. Try it. You will be delighted with the result.

17.2 THE CREATIVE IMAGINATION (CHAPTER V)

The Process of Creative Imagination

THERE is another type of imagination from the purely reproductive memory imagination of which we have been speaking in this book.

There is also Creative Imagination.

Creative Imagination is more than mere memory. It takes the elements of the past as reproduced by memory and rearranges them. It forms new combinations out of the material of the past. It forms new combinations of ideas, emotions and their accompanying impulses to muscular activity, the elements of mental "complexes." It recombines these elements into new and original mental pictures, the creations of the inventive mind.

Business and Financial Imagination

No particular profession or pursuit has a monopoly of creative imagination. It is not the exclusive property of the poet, the artist, the inventor, the philosopher. We tell you this because you have heard all your life of the poetic imagination, the artistic imagination, and so on, but it is rare indeed that you have heard mention of the business imagination.

The fact is no man can succeed in any pursuit unless he has a creative imagination. Without creative imagination the human race would still be living in caves. Without creative imagination there would be no ships, no engines, no automobiles, no corporations, no systems, no plans, no business. Nothing exists in all the world that had not a previous counterpart in the mind of him who designed it. And back of all is the creative mind of God.

How Wealth is Created

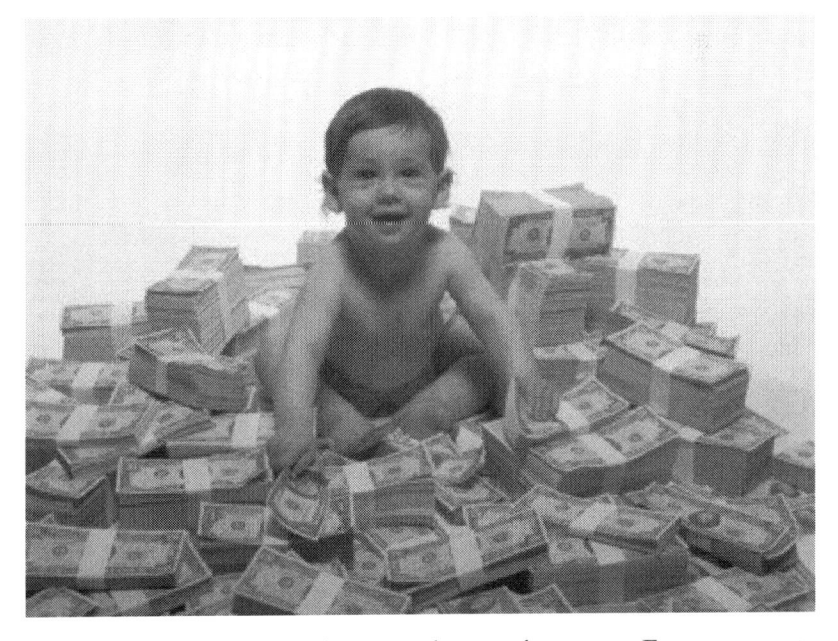

Mind is supreme. Mind shapes and controls matter. Every concrete thing in the world is the product of a thinking consciousness. The richly tinted canvas is the physical expression of the artist's dream. The great factory, with its whirling mechanisms and glowing furnaces, is the material manifestation of the promoter's financial imagination. The jewelled ornament, the book, the steamship, the office building, all are but concrete realizations of human thought moulded out of formless matter.

Mind, finite and infinite, is eternally creative and creating in the organization of formless matter and material forces into concrete realities.

The Klamath Philosophy

Says Max Müller in his "Psychological Religion": "The Klamaths, one of the Red Indian tribes, believe in a Supreme God whom they call 'The Most Ancient One,' 'Our Old Father,' or 'The Old One on High.' He is believed to have created the world—that is, to have made plants, animals and man. But when asked how the Old Father created the world, the Klamath philosopher replies: *'By thinking and willing.'*"

How Men Get Things

We get what we desire because the things we desire are the things we think about. Love begets love. The man who is looking for trouble generally finds it. Despair is the forerunner of disaster, and fear brings failure, because despair and fear are the emotional elements attendant upon thoughts of defeat.

Behind every thing and every act is, and always has been, thought—thought of sufficient intensity to shape and fashion the physical event.

Mind, and mind alone, possesses the inscrutable power to create.

Your career is ordered by the thoughts you entertain. Mental pictures tend to accomplish their own realization. Therefore, be careful to hold only those thoughts that will build up rather than tear down the structure of your fortunes.

Prerequisites to Achievement

Creative imagination is an absolute prerequisite to material achievement.

The business man must scheme and plan and devise and foresee. He must create in imagination today the results that he is to achieve tomorrow. He must combine the elements of his past experiential complexes into a mental picture of future events as he would have them. Riches are but the material realization of a financial imagination. The wealth of the world is but the sum total of the contributions of the creative thoughts of the successful men of all ages.

How to Take Radical Steps in Business

With these principles before you, you can plainly see that the *creative imagination must be called upon in the solution of every practical question in every hour of the business day.*

Consider its part in two phases of your business life—first, when you are contemplating a radical change in your business situation; second, when you are seeking to improve some particular department of your business.

How to Take Radical Steps in Business

In the determination of how best you can better yourself, either in your present field of action or by the selection of a new one, take the following steps: (1) Pass in review before the mind's eye your present situation; (2) Your possible ways of betterment; (3) The various circumstances and individuals that will aid in this or that line of self-advancement; (4) The difficulties that may confront you. Having selected your field, (5) Consider various possible plans of action; (6) Have prevision of their working out; (7) Compare the ultimate results as you foresee them; (8) Decide upon the one most promising, and then with this plan as a foundation for further imaginings, (9) Once more call before you the elements that will contribute to success; (10) See the possible locations for your new place of business and choose among them; (11) Outline in detail the methods to be pursued in getting and handling business; (12) See the different kinds of employees and associates you will require, and select certain classes as best suited to your needs; (13) Foresee possible difficulties to be encountered and adjust your plans to meet them; and, most important of all, (14) Have a clear and persistent vision of yourself as a man of action, setting to work upon your plan at a fixed hour and carrying it to a successful issue within a given time.

The Expansion of Business Ideals

There is excellent practical psychology in the following from "Thoughts on Business":

"Men often think of a position as being just about so big and no bigger, when, as a matter of fact, a position is often what one makes it. A man was making about $1,500 a year out of a certain position and thought he was doing all that could be done to advance the business. The employer thought otherwise, and gave the place to another man who soon made the position worth $8,000 a year—at exactly the same commission.

Rising to the Emergency

"The difference was in the men—in other words, in what the two men thought about the work. One had a little conception of what the work should be, and the other had a big conception of it. One thought little thoughts, and the other thought big thoughts.

"The standards of two men may differ, not especially because one is naturally more capable than the other, but because one is familiar with big things and the other is not. The time was when the former worked in a smaller scope himself, but when he saw a wider view of what his work might be he rose to the occasion and became a bigger man. It is just as easy to think of a mountain as to think of a hill—when you turn your mind to contemplate it. The mind is like a rubber band—you can stretch it to fit almost anything, but it draws in to a small scope when you let go.

The Constructive Imagination

"Make it your business to know what is the best that might be in your line of work, and stretch your mind to conceive it, and then devise some way to attain it.

Little Tasks and Big Tasks

"Big things are only little things put together. I was greatly impressed with this fact one morning as I stood watching the workmen erecting the steel framework for a tall office building. A shrill whistle rang out as a signal, a man over at the engine pulled a lever, a chain from the derrick was lowered, and the whistle rang out again. A man stooped down and fastened the chain around the centre of a steel beam, stepped back and blew the whistle once more. Again the lever was moved at the engine, and the steel beam soared into the air up to the sixteenth story, where it was made fast by little bolts.

"The entire structure, great as it was, towering far above all the neighbouring buildings, was made up of pieces of steel and stone and wood, put together according to a plan. The plan was first imagined, then pencilled, then carefully drawn, and then followed by the workmen. It was all a combination of little things.

Working Up a Department

"It is encouraging to think of this when you are confronted by a big task. Remember that it is only a group of little tasks, any of which you can easily do. It is ignorance of this fact that makes some men afraid to try."

Suppose, now, that instead of making a radical change in your business situation, you are simply seeking to improve some particular department of your business.

Imagination in Handling Employees

In commercial affairs men are the great means to money-making, and efficient personal service the great key to prosperity. In your dealings with employees do not be guided by the necessities of the moment. Expediency is the poorest of all excuses for action. Have regard not only for your own immediate needs, but also for the welfare and future conduct of your employees. It is part of the burden of the executive head that he must do the fore thinking not only for himself but for those under him.

Perhaps the man you have under observation for advancement to some executive position has all the basic qualifications of judicial sense, discrimination and attentiveness to details, but you are uncertain whether he has enough imagination to devise new ways and means of doing things and developing business in new fields. If you wish to try a simple but very effective test along this line, you can adopt the following standard psychological experiment, which has been used at Harvard, Cornell and many other colleges and schools.

How to Test an Employee's Imagination

Let fall a drop of ink on each of several pieces of white paper, letterhead size. This will make irregular blotches of varying forms. Let the subject be seated at a desk and ask him to write briefly about what he sees in each blotched sheet, whether it be an animal form suggested by the outline of the blot, or anything else that comes into his mind while looking at the black spot. The principle involved here is the same as that involved in seeing pictures in a flickering log fire or having a vision of past or future events by gazing into a crystal. In any of these cases, it is not the blot, the fire or the crystal that produces the vision, but the creative imagination that recombines old elements into new forms. The number of images suggested to one by certain standard forms of ink-blot when compared with established results is a measure of his imaginative ability.

Imagination in Business Generally

In the choice of a location for your factory or store, you must foresee its future traffic and transportation possibilities. In passing upon a proposed advertisement you must get inside the head of the man on the street and see it as he will see it. In the purchase of your stock of goods you must gauge the trend of popular taste and foresee the big demand. In your dealings with creditors you must plan a course of action that will enable you to settle the account to *your* best interest at *their* request. You must find a way to collect from your debtors and at the same time hold their business. And so in a hundred thousand different ways you are constantly required to use creative thought in laying every stone in the structure of your fortune.

Imagination and Action

Do not understand us as saying that imagination, as the term is popularly used, is all you need. There must be also action, incessant, persistent. But *creative imagination, in a psychological and scientific sense, begets action. Every thought carries with it the impellent energy to effect its realization.* Use your imagination in your business and the action will take care of itself. Given imagination and action, and you are sure to win.

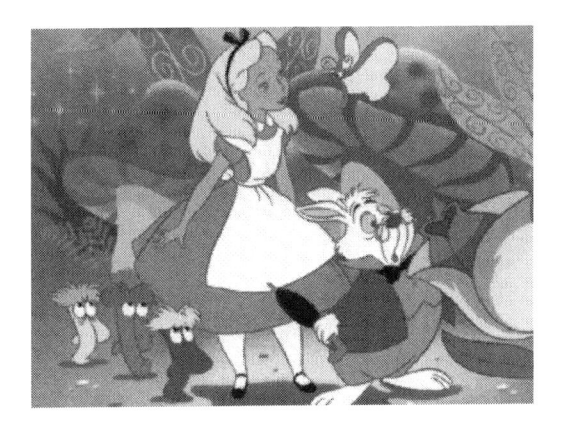

THANK YOU

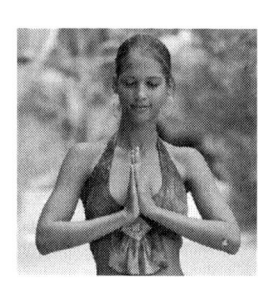

I hope you enjoyed the book

Check for more books of Dean Amory at:

http://www.lulu.com/spotlight/Jaimelavie

Manufactured by Amazon.ca
Bolton, ON